The Art of

Natural
Family
Planning®

Postpartum
Student Guide

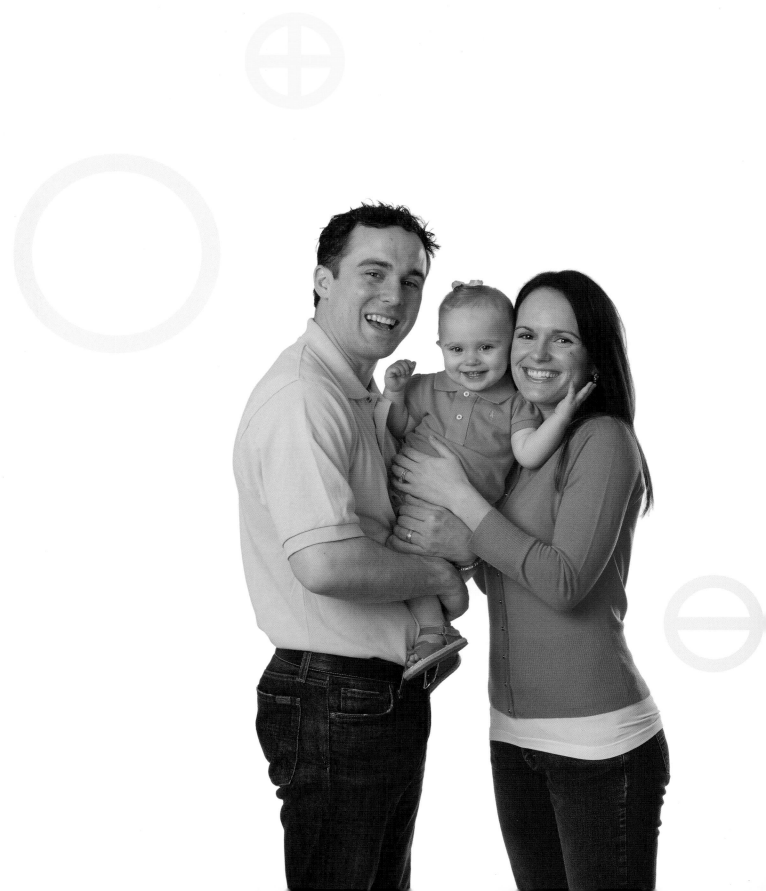

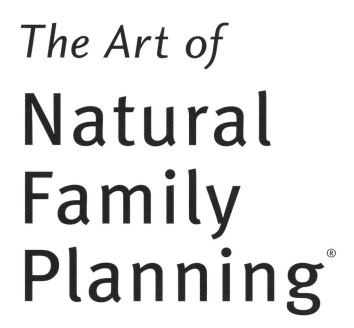

The Art of
Natural Family Planning®

Postpartum
Student Guide

The Couple to Couple League
International, Inc.
P.O. Box 111184
Cincinnati, OH 45211-1184

This text is an integral part of The Couple to Couple League's (CCL) natural family planning instructional course, specifically, the Postpartum Class. Natural family planning is best learned through a class series taught by a certified CCL Teacher or through CCL's Home Study Program. For information on how to get in touch with a CCL certified teacher, visit the CCL website at **www.ccli.org.**

Book Design by Scott Bruno of b graphic design
Cover Photo by Ron Rack of Rack Photography

Cataloging data
        L.C. 2008941156

The Art of Natural Family Planning® Postpartum Student Guide
The Couple to Couple League
Natural Family Planning
Birth Control
Breastfeeding
Sexual Morality

ISBN 978-0-926412-32-3

Published by The Couple to Couple League International, Inc.
P.O. Box 111184
Cincinnati, OH 45211
U.S.A.
800-745-8252
www.ccli.org

Printed in the United States
10 9 8 7 6 5 4 3 2 1

Table of Contents

Preface P

Most users of Natural Family Planning (NFP) will agree that when a woman's fertility is in a state of transition — like following the birth of a baby — it can cause a degree of uncertainty and less confidence in their ability to effectively assess their fertility. Many couples

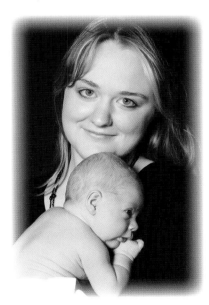

contact The Couple to Couple League with questions during these times. Our experience has been that we have watched their confidence grow as they gain information about what is happening hormonally during this time of transition.

For this reason, CCL is very excited about the publication of this manual, which focuses on the practice of the Sympto-Thermal Method of NFP during the postpartum time. *The Art of Natural Family Planning® Postpartum Student Guide* accompanies CCL's new class dedicated solely to this time of transition, which is available to any couple taking the main NFP course who happens to be in, or approaching, the postpartum transition. In addition, current members who have learned NFP from CCL in the past, but who are now in need of this specialized information, are also welcome to take this class if they have already learned the new methodology in CCL's current NFP program (released in January 2008).

More knowledge empowers people, and it is our hope that this new manual and CCL's new Postpartum Class will help NFP couples have greater confidence in their ability to effectively navigate the transition from birth to the return of regular fertility cycles.

Introduction 1

The Postpartum Class is divided into seven lessons: *Introduction, Review, The Postpartum Woman, The Benefits of Breastfeeding, Baby Feeding and Fertility, Fertility Awareness after Childbirth,* and *Postpartum Decisions: NFP and Responsible Parenthood.* This *Introduction* will summarize the Postpartum lessons.

Summary: Postpartum Class Lessons

Lesson 2, *Review*, uses a practice chart to discuss the concepts taught in Classes 1 and 2 of CCL's main Natural Family Planning course, emphasizing the Phase I rules and the Sympto-Thermal Rule (ST Rule). This knowledge is necessary to understand the transition from pregnancy to the return of fertility after childbirth.

Lesson 3, *The Postpartum Woman*, explains how the reproductive hormones function after childbirth in a way that can delay ovulation. This lesson also discusses possible concerns women may have after delivery and strategies for a good postpartum recovery, including the importance of good nutrition, especially during the first six weeks postpartum.

In the lesson *The Benefits of Breastfeeding*, you will learn the many advantages of breast-feeding and how it provides the best nutrition for baby, assists mothers in recovering from childbirth, and promotes a natural bond between mother and baby. In addition, you will see how breastfeeding can benefit the entire family, and why it is recommended by both national and international organizations for a minimum of 12 months, and longer if possible.

Lesson 5, *Baby Feeding and Fertility*, defines the various types of baby feeding and briefly discusses how each one can affect the return of fertility after childbirth.

Lesson 6, *Fertility Awareness after Childbirth*, explains how to read and interpret your signs of fertility as your body is adjusting to the changing hormones after childbirth. This lesson will delineate when to begin observing and recording the key measurable signs of fertility — cervical mucus, temperature, and the cervix — whether your baby is formula-fed (bottle-fed) or breastfed.

As you learned in Class 2, married love should be modeled after the five characteristics of divine love. Each spouse must *choose to give* himself or herself to the other based on the *knowledge* of their value and dignity as persons made in the image and likeness of God. This *self-gift* must be *permanent* and *life-giving*. With this in mind, the last lesson, *Postpartum Decisions: NFP and Responsible Parenthood*, initiates a discussion regarding marital intimacy (which is broader than sexual intimacy) and responsible parenthood (the virtuous decision to plan or to postpone a pregnancy).

The Postpartum Class will help you to:

- Recognize the hormonal changes as your body transitions from pregnancy to your pre-pregnancy reproductive cycles
- Appreciate the many benefits of breastfeeding
- Know the various types of baby feeding and how each one can affect your return of fertility
- Learn how to apply NFP during the postpartum time
- Make informed decisions regarding future pregnancies

Notes

Review 2

Lesson 2

This *Review* will ensure that you can properly identify the three phases of the menstrual cycle, and know when and how to apply the Phase I Guidelines and Rules and the Sympto-Thermal Rule (ST Rule). This foundation in the Sympto-Thermal Method of NFP will bring you confidence in reading and interpreting the signs of fertility during the postpartum transition.

Phase I Guidelines and Rules

In previous classes, you learned that Phase I begins on the first day of menstruation, and Phase II begins with the onset of fertility signs. Phase I is usually distinguished by the absence of cervical mucus sensations and characteristics, and by a drop in the basal body temperature to the pre-ovulation levels of previous cycles. The presence of mucus is a fundamental condition for defining the start of Phase II, the fertile time.

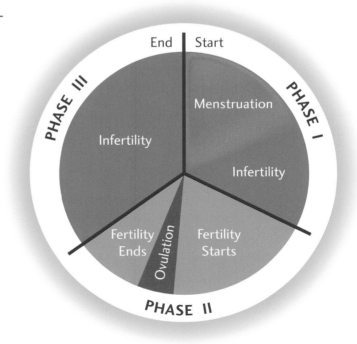

Phase III is the time of infertility beginning several days after ovulation and continuing until the next menstruation.

When applying the rules to determine the limits of Phase I infertility, it is important to follow the two basic guidelines. Once menstruation decreases:

- Limit marital relations to the evenings of dry/nothing mucus days during Phase I.

- Abstain on any day that follows marital relations in Phase I unless you are experienced and can positively detect the absence of mucus.

The Phase I rules are summarized in this lesson. However, for a more detailed explanation, see *The Art of Natural Family Planning® Student Guide*, Class 2, Lesson 4, *The Transition from Phase I to Phase II*, pages 77–87, or the Reference Guide, *Rules Summary*, pages 261–263.

Last Dry Day Rule

This rule requires at least six cycles of experience observing and recording cervical mucus signs.
- The end of Phase I is the last day without mucus sensations or characteristics.

Shortest-Cycle Rule

The following principles assume the absence of cervical mucus.

- *Women with cycles 26 days or longer* in the last 12 cycles can assume infertility on Cycle Days 1 through 6.

- *Women with at least one cycle less than 26 days* in the last 12 cycles can assume infertility on the cycle days preceding and including their previous shortest cycle minus 20.

- *Women with no knowledge of their previous cycle history* can assume infertility on Cycle Days 1 through 5 until they have 12 cycles of history. If they experience a subsequent cycle that is less than 26 days long, they can assume infertility on the cycle days preceding and including the shortest cycle minus 20.

- *Women who have recently discontinued the birth control pill or patch, or other non-injectable hormonal birth control,* can assume infertility on Cycle Days 1 through 5 until they have 12 cycles of history. They should wait three full menstrual cycles before applying this rule. If they experience a subsequent cycle that is less than 26 days long, they can assume infertility on the cycle days preceding and including the shortest cycle minus 20.

Doering Rule

This rule assumes the absence of mucus and requires six cycles of temperature history.

- Subtract seven from the earliest first day of temperature rise in the last 12 cycles.[1] Mark that cycle day as the last day that you can assume Phase I infertility.

Phase III: The Sympto-Thermal (ST) Rule:

Phase III begins on the evening of:

1. The third day of drying-up after Peak Day, combined with

2. Three normal post-peak temperatures in a rising pattern above the LTL

AND the third temperature at or above the HTL
OR the cervix closed and hard for three days

If the above conditions are not met, then Phase III begins after waiting an additional post-peak day for another temperature above the LTL.

(To review the steps for applying the ST Rule, see the Appendix, page 54.)

Notes

---

[1] Women who have less than 12 cycles of temperature history can use this rule if they have *at least six cycles* of temperature history.

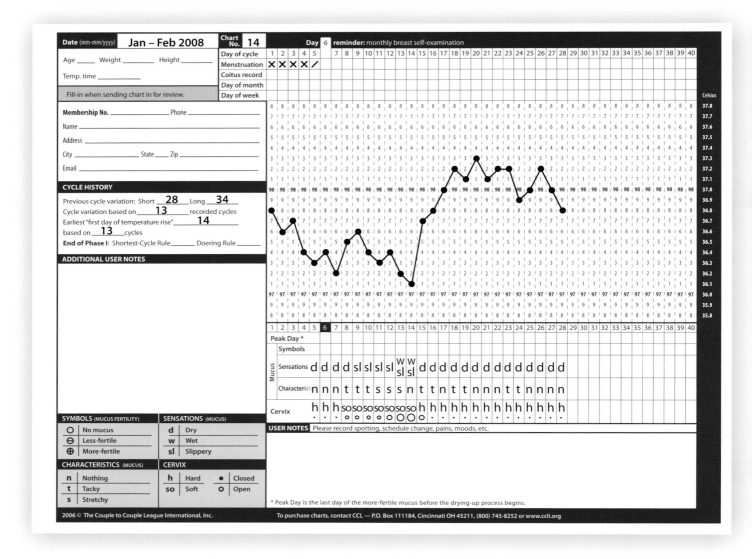

If you are attending the Postpartum Class, you will complete this exercise in class. If you are using this Postpartum Student Guide on your own, be sure to check your answers on page 55 of the Appendix.

1. Apply a mucus symbol for Cycle Days 5 through 28 on the chart: $\bigcirc, \ominus, \oplus$.

2. Determine the end of Phase I by calculating:

   - Shortest-Cycle Rule (Circle the appropriate day and record it in the correct box.)

   - Doering Rule (Circle the appropriate day and record it in the correct box.)

   - Last Dry Day Rule

3. Draw a vertical line between Phase I and Phase II indicating the latest possible end of Phase I.

4. Determine the first day of Phase III by applying the ST Rule. Draw a vertical line through the temperature and circle that cycle day on the chart.

Be sure you understand how to properly analyze the review chart in this lesson before moving on to the next lesson. The Postpartum Class assumes that you understand Classes 1 and 2 of the main CCL course in Natural Family Planning. If you have any questions, contact a local CCL Teaching Couple or the main office for assistance.[2]

Notes

---

[2] NFP consulting is free for those who have received instruction from CCL (class series or Home Study Course) **and** have a current CCL membership. Others may receive consulting help for a fee.

3 The Postpartum Woman

Lesson 3

Postpartum is the term used to explain that a mother has recently given birth and has not yet returned to her pre-pregnancy state. During this time, a mother will experience a variety of physical, psychological, physiological, and perhaps even spiritual changes as she transitions from nurturing her baby in utero to nurturing him or her after birth.

You may recall how the four key reproductive hormones interact during a woman's non-pregnant fertile years. The pituitary gland releases Follicle Stimulating Hormone (FSH). This hormone increases during Phase I in order to stimulate immature eggs within the follicles (the egg sacs) to develop into mature eggs. As the follicle develops, it produces estrogen, and as the estrogen increases, it causes observable changes in the cervical mucus and cervix in preparation for ovulation. Luteinizing Hormone (LH), another chemical messenger, is also released by the pituitary gland. During Phase I, LH rises slightly, but maintains a relatively low level until right before ovulation. At that time the pituitary gland quickly produces a large amount of LH, which signals the release of the mature egg (**ovulation**) into the Fallopian tube.

During pregnancy, **prolactin** (called "the mothering hormone") increases significantly and aids in the accelerated growth of the breast tissue,[3] which is why a woman's breasts contain

---

[3] Thomas W. Hilgers, M.D. *Reproductive Anatomy & Physiology*, Second edition (December 2002), 46.

fluid during the second half of her pregnancy. After a woman delivers a baby and the **placenta** (the organ inside the uterus that supplies food and oxygen to, and removes wastes from, the unborn baby through the umbilical cord), the hormones estrogen and progesterone abruptly drop. The decrease in these two hormones helps stimulate the release of more prolactin from the pituitary gland; from this point, prolactin levels are dependent on milk removal and breastfeeding. With **suckling** (feeding from the breast), prolactin levels increase, and the hormone continues to stimulate and maintain the secretion of milk. Prolactin enables natural bonding between mother and baby that begins early in pregnancy, maximizes near delivery, and then continues with the baby's suckling. The suckling also releases another hormone, **oxytocin**, which facilitates the let-down of milk during nursing and assists in this postpartum bonding.

As the pituitary gland increases its production of prolactin, it suppresses its production of LH. As long as LH remains low, ovulation is delayed, thus causing a time of natural infertility. This is called **lactational amenorrhea** (lack of menstrual periods due to breastfeeding). Breastfeeding, therefore, can greatly affect the length of lactational amenorrhea because it stimulates the production of prolactin and suppresses the hormones that are necessary for ovulation. On the other hand, non-breastfeeding mothers usually experience a much shorter time of postpartum infertility — perhaps three weeks or more.

For about five weeks after childbirth, she produces a blood-tinged discharge called **lochia**. Lochia is heavy at first, but gradually tapers off. When her cycles return, a postpartum woman will usually have a longer length of time between menstruations, with her cycles gradually returning to their pre-pregnancy length.

Possible Concerns during Recovery

As you can see, there is much going on hormonally in a woman's body during both the immediate postpartum days and weeks, and even longer if she breastfeeds her baby. While you may feel you have reached the end of a journey as you hold your precious newborn in your arms, you still have significant paths to travel: adjusting to motherhood (either for the first time, or with a new addition to the family), and physically recovering from the birth. It is good to be aware of some of the difficulties you may encounter in the early weeks and months.

Notes

Rapidly changing levels of hormones following the birth, as well as the physically demanding birth itself, can lead to new mothers experiencing several, or even all, of the following:

- Cramping

- Constipation

- Hemorrhoids

- Vaginal pain

- Postpartum urinary incontinence

- Hair loss

- Exhaustion

- Postpartum blues

- Postpartum depression

Fortunately, many of these occurrences are minor, easily handled, and tend to resolve themselves within a few weeks. This lesson will briefly discuss each of these experiences and offer strategies that may help to alleviate them.

Strategies for a Good Recovery[4]

Cramping: The uterus continues to contract in the weeks after the birth in order to return to its normal size. These contractions also help slow, and eventually stop, the postpartum bleeding by closing off tiny blood vessels in the uterine lining. Over the early postpartum weeks, these contractions may feel similar to menstrual cramps, and may be more noticeable if you are breastfeeding, as the baby's suckling releases the hormone oxytocin. In addition to stimulating milk let-down, oxytocin contracts the uterus. If the discomfort (which can last up to six weeks) is more than mild or interferes with your breastfeeding, ask your doctor about pain relievers that are safe for you to take as a breastfeeding mother.

Constipation: Difficulty with bowel movements following birth is to be expected for several reasons, such as trauma to rectal (sphincter) muscles during delivery, or increased levels of progesterone, which slows digestion and the passage of food through the intestines. This is a good time to focus on drinking plenty of water and obtaining a healthy amount of fiber through eating fruits, vegetables, and whole grains. If your doctor permits, mild exercise may also help.

---

[4] Information in this section was compiled primarily from William Sears, M.D. and Martha Sears, R.N., *The Baby Book* (New York: Little, Brown and Company, 2003), and William Sears, M.D. and Martha Sears, R.N., *The Pregnancy Book* (New York: Little, Brown and Company, 1997).

Hemorrhoids: Many women find that if hemorrhoids did not develop during the later months of pregnancy, they resulted from the pushing and straining of the delivery. Focusing on nutrition (and especially fiber intake) is important here as well, since you will want to try to avoid constipation. If your hemorrhoids are tender, warm sitz baths may help. Talk to your doctor if you have any concerns about their healing.

Vaginal pain: You can expect to have a sore and tender perineum for a time after giving birth, due to the stretching and stress in this area. Some women are unable to avoid an episiotomy, and will have stitches and a sore incision; others experience some minor tearing that needs to heal. Heat (warmth) promotes blood flow and promotes healing; therefore, warm (not hot) sitz baths are recommended. Cold decreases swelling and numbs the area, and thus ice packs can provide relief. Also, pay attention to personal cleanliness to help avoid infection. If healing is slow, or if you experience any sharp pains in your vagina, talk to your doctor.

Postpartum urinary incontinence: It is not unusual to experience temporary **urinary incontinence** (the inability to keep urine in the bladder) during the early weeks after childbirth. This is caused by the bladder muscles being stretched during late pregnancy and the delivery. As your organs and muscles return to their pre-pregnancy position, any incontinence should resolve itself. In the meantime, wear a pantiliner if necessary, and talk to your doctor if this has not cleared up by your postpartum checkup.

Hair loss: In the early weeks after childbirth, many women report that their hair seems to be falling out. In reality, the pregnancy hormones prevented the normal shedding of hair, and as your hormone levels return to normal, hair loss may simply seem excessive. No treatment is necessary.

Exhaustion: This is one postpartum occurrence that is probably universal. As your body has likely been through the most strenuous work of your life, you can expect to feel a level of exhaustion that you have never experienced before, as well as feeling achy and stiff for awhile. There is no better strategy than to rest as much as possible, and try to sleep whenever the baby sleeps. Rely on others for household assistance, and try not to worry about the work that may need to be done. Focus instead on your healing and on your baby.

Postpartum blues: Many mothers are surprised to experience "weepiness" or sadness in the early days and weeks after giving birth, but for 50–75% of mothers[5] this is actually a normal experience that results from hormonal fluctuations. You may also experience mood swings, crying, anxiety, impatience, lack of concentration, etc. These symptoms are usually mild and disappear in a few weeks. Be sure to get plenty of rest, concentrate on your recovery, and rely on others for household help.

---

[5] William Sears, M.D. and Martha Sears, R.N., *The Baby Book* (New York: Little, Brown and Company, 2003) 65.

Postpartum depression: For 10–20% of mothers, the postpartum blues may develop into postpartum depression,[6] although postpartum depression (PPD) can also begin at any time during the first year. This can manifest itself as excessive fatigue, insomnia, changes in appetite, difficulty in making decisions, feeling hopeless, negative attitudes, and even thoughts of death or suicide. While PPD can be troubling, it is usually highly treatable, so be sure to talk to your doctor about what you are experiencing. (It is interesting to note that the higher levels of prolactin and oxytocin help decrease anxiety and are physiologically soothing to a breastfeeding mother.)

Nutritional Support

In order to minimize difficulties or promote healing from many of these postpartum occurrences, good nutrition is very important, especially during the first six weeks post-partum. You should strive for a balanced diet of protein, complex carbohydrates (such as fresh fruits and vegetables), and healthy fats. Avoid trans-saturated (partially-hydrogenated or hydrogenated) fats and empty calories (such as sugary or pre-sweetened products), and be sure to include healthy essential fatty acids through certified toxin-free fish oils, cod liver oil, flaxseed oil, or healthy fish.[7] Many doctors recommend taking a vitamin/mineral supplement that includes calcium. If you have not already done so, you may want to discuss this with your doctor.

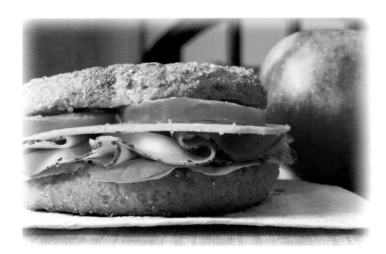

Notes

---

[6] Sears and Sears, 66.

[7] Toxin-free fish oils, including cod liver oil, are readily available at health food stores. For further information, see *Fertility, Cycles & Nutrition,* Fourth edition, and the National Resource Defense Council website: *www.nrdc.org/health/effects/mercury/guide.asp*

The Benefits of Breastfeeding[8]

4

Lesson 4

Breastfeeding provides the best nutrition for babies. In fact, breastfeeding is so important that the American Academy of Pediatrics (AAP) provides an extensive set of instructions for pediatricians and other health care professionals to protect, promote, and support breastfeeding, "…not only in their individual practices but also in the hospital, medical school, community, and nation."[9] The AAP even goes so far as to challenge these experts to provide advice to adoptive mothers who decide to breastfeed through **induced lactation** (the process by which a non-pregnant mother is stimulated to **lactate** — produce milk).

Why is there such remarkable support for breastfeeding from this prestigious organization? The answer lies in the opening sentence of the "2005 AAP Policy Statement of Breastfeeding and the Use of Human Milk": "Considerable advances have occurred in recent years in the scientific knowledge of the benefits of breastfeeding, the mechanisms underlying these benefits, and in the clinical management of breastfeeding."

These benefits are not specific only to babies; breastfeeding promotes natural bonding between mother and baby through the combined action of the hormones prolactin and

---

[8] This lesson will discuss several of the benefits of breastfeeding; however, it is not intended to be an exhaustive analysis of this topic. For further information, see the documents referenced in this lesson and Class 3, Lesson 8, *Benefits of Breastfeeding and Its Effect on Fertility*, pp. 153–162 in *The Art of Natural Family Planning® Student Guide*, and *The Art of Breastfeeding* by Linda Kracht and Jackie Hilgert (Cincinnati: The Couple to Couple League, 2008).

[9] "2005 AAP Policy Statement of Breastfeeding and the Use of Human Milk," *Pediatrics*, Vol. 115, No. 2 (February 2005) 496.

oxytocin (discussed earlier in this class). Oxytocin helps decrease anxiety and increases a mother's attention to her baby. Later in this lesson, you will also see how breastfeeding assists mothers in recovering from childbirth, and how it can benefit the entire family.

To maximize these benefits, several eminent organizations have joined the AAP in advocating **exclusive breastfeeding**[10] for the first six months of an infant's life. Among these organizations are the American College of Obstetricians and Gynecologists (ACOG), the American Academy of Family Physicians, the Academy of Breastfeeding Medicine (ABM), the World Health Organization (WHO), the United Nation's Children's Fund, and several other health organizations.[11] Furthermore, the American Academy of Pediatrics (AAP) recommends continued breastfeeding as the standard of care for all babies for a minimum of 12 months, and the WHO recommends breastfeeding for a minimum of 24 months.[12] The Couple to Couple League also advocates exclusive breastfeeding and promotes continued breastfeeding with baby-led weaning. The various types of baby feeding are more clearly defined in Lesson 5, *Baby Feeding and Fertility*, pages 17–20.

Benefits of Breastfeeding › Baby

Breastfeeding enhances a child's overall health. In the United States, post-neonatal infant mortality rates are reduced by 21% in breastfed babies.[13] Following delivery, a yellowish liquid called **colostrum** is secreted by a mother's breasts for about the first three to five days. This powerful substance is different from human breast milk. Colostrum is rich in **antibodies** (proteins that fight infections), and it contains more protein and minerals, and less sugar and fat, than human breast milk. It is interesting to note that a mother's milk is biologically and immunologically appropriate for her baby, even if the baby is born prematurely. In addition, breast milk provides both primary and secondary protection against viral, bacterial, and allergic diseases.[14]

---

[10] 2005 AAP Policy Statement, 498. "Exclusive breastfeeding is defined as an infant's consumption of human milk with no supplementation of any type (no water, no juice, no nonhuman milk, and no foods) except for vitamins, minerals, and medications."

[11] Ibid.

[12] J. Lauwers and A. Swisher, *Counseling the Nursing Mother, A Lactation Consultant's Guide*, 2005, 167; *Pediatrics*, Vol. 115, No. 2, February 2005, 496-506; World Health Organization, *Infant and young child nutrition: Global strategy on infant and young child feeding*, Fifty-fifth World Health Assembly, 16 April 2002.

[13] 2005 AAP Policy Statement, 496.

[14] Jon Weimer, *The Economic Benefits of Breastfeeding* (Economic Research Service/USDA, 2001) 10.

Breastfeeding also acts as an analgesic during a painful procedure (such as a heel stick on a newborn), and cognitive development studies show better performance in breastfed babies compared to formula-fed infants.[15] Furthermore, the AAP cites studies that suggest "decreased rates of sudden infant death syndrome [SIDS] in the first year of life and reduction in incidence of insulin-dependent (type 1) and non-insulin-dependent (type 2) diabetes mellitus, lymphoma, leukemia, and Hodgkin's disease, overweight and obesity, hypercholesterolemia, and asthma in older children and adults who were breastfed, compared with individuals who were not breastfed."[16]

Benefits of Breastfeeding › Mother

Breastfeeding provides significant health benefits for a mother as well as for her newborn. In the previous lesson, you learned that the hormone oxytocin, released during breastfeeding, is responsible for producing the let-down reflex that makes breast milk

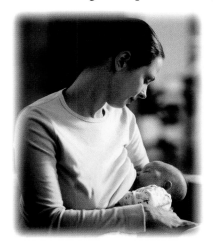 available to the baby. This same hormone also causes the uterine muscles to contract, which decreases postpartum bleeding and enables the uterus to return to its pre-pregnancy size. Because oxytocin is so beneficial for decreasing postpartum blood loss, most doctors and midwives encourage mothers to breastfeed their newborns immediately after giving birth. (In addition, newborns are usually most alert and show readiness to breastfeed at this time.)

There are several other advantages for mothers who nurse their babies. Many women appreciate that it causes an earlier return to their pre-pregnancy weight. It has also been known to decrease the risks of breast and ovarian cancers, and possibly even to decrease the risk of hip fractures and osteoporosis in postmenopausal women who breastfed their babies.[17]

Along with all of these other significant advantages, mothers who breastfeed will usually enjoy a time of postpartum infertility, depending largely on how often the baby nurses, how many weeks or months the nursing continues, and the mother's individual physiology. This time of natural infertility is an opportunity for a mother to recover from the pregnancy and delivery. The length of time between the birth of a baby and the return of fertility depends on many factors. (These will be discussed in the next lesson.) However, it

---

[15] 2005 AAP Policy Statement, 497.

[16] 2005 AAP Policy Statement, 496–497.

[17] 2005 AAP Policy Statement, 497.

is important to note that there is strong evidence that confirms the relative infertility of *the first six months after childbirth while exclusively breastfeeding and experiencing lactational amenorrhea.*[18]

Benefits of Breastfeeding › Family

Breastfeeding can cause a positive chain reaction within a family: The infant receives sound nutrition and comfort when he nurses; the mother acquires short term and long term health benefits; and more time can be devoted to other family members because of decreased infant illness and the fact that the baby's food is always ready — no preparation time needs to be factored into the family's schedule.

In addition, the family saves an average of $900–$1,200 yearly in the United States[19] that would otherwise be spent on formula. Furthermore, in its discussion of the benefits of breastfeeding, the AAP includes "the potential for decreased annual health care costs of $3.6 *billion* [emphasis added] in the United States…and decreased parental employee absenteeism and associated loss of income…"[20]

Notes

---

[18] See Lesson 5, *Baby Feeding and Fertility*, pages 19–20.

[19] Lauwers and Swisher, 177.

[20] 2005 AAP Policy Statement, 497.

Baby Feeding and Fertility 5

Lesson 5

After childbirth, most mothers will experience at least three weeks, and usually several more, during which they are infertile. This absence of fertility results in a subsequent absence of menstrual periods — **amenorrhea**. **Lactating** (breastfeeding, milk producing) mothers will normally experience a longer length of amenorrhea than **non-lactating** (non-breastfeeding, formula feeding) mothers. For many years, however, family planning and lactation experts observed that the length of this lactational amenorrhea varied greatly among breastfeeding mothers. Further research led to the identification of several key factors that, combined with a woman's own physiology, influence the length of amenorrhea while breastfeeding. These factors include:

- **Duration** (the number of months)

- **Frequency** (the number of feeds within 24 hours), and

- **Intensity** (influenced by the use or non-use of bottles, pacifiers, solid foods, and other factors).

In this lesson you will learn about the four types of baby feeding — formula feeding, mixed breastfeeding, exclusive breastfeeding, and continued breastfeeding — and how each one can affect the return of fertility after childbirth.

Formula Feeding

Formula feeding means that a baby is fed with a bottle and receives only formula, ranging from cow's milk to specialty formulas. Typically, there is an early return of fertility postpartum: usually ranging from seven to nine weeks. (Note that while donated breast milk is not considered formula, couples who choose to feed their babies donated breast milk should use the return of fertility instructions associated with formula feeding.)

Breastfeeding

Mixed breastfeeding (or **mixed feeding**) is a combination of formula and/or pumped breast milk and breastfeeding. **High mixed breastfeeding** means that 80% of the feeding comes from the breast. **Medium mixed breastfeeding** means that 20–79% of the feeding is from the breast, and **low mixed breastfeeding** occurs when less than 20% of the feeding comes from the breast. Mixed breastfeeding may also include a combination of breastfeeding, bottles, and early introduction of solids. It can also mean that a baby nurses according to a schedule, or uses a pacifier[21] regularly, limiting the amount of time that he suckles.

Baby Feeding & Fertility

Mixed Breastfeeding

- **High**
  80% of feeding is from the breast

- **Medium**
  20–79% of feeding is from the breast

- **Low**
  Less than 20% of feeding is from the breast

Mixed breastfeeding may delay ovulation, but the return of fertility varies greatly, depending on the amount of suckling (i.e., duration, frequency, and intensity) and the mother's physiology. It is important to note that mixed breastfeeding will usually lead to an earlier return of fertility because the baby breastfeeds less frequently.

---

[21] 2005 AAP Policy Statement, 499. The AAP recommends avoiding pacifier use until breastfeeding is well established.

Exclusive breastfeeding is defined as nursing whenever the baby indicates a desire (day or night) *during his first six months of life.*[22] The baby derives all of his nutrition from the breast, and he receives no bottles or early solids. The baby stays near his mother so that he can nurse and pacify at the breast on his own schedule; he does not regularly use a pacifier.

Generally, mothers who exclusively breastfeed are highly infertile during this time. Much of this evidence was gathered at a conference held in Bellagio, Italy in 1988.[23] Family planning experts from around the world tracked the return of fertility in mothers who were not using any method of family planning or fertility awareness while they were *exclusively breastfeeding.* Their findings revealed significant infertility in the first 56 days (eight weeks) postpartum, and less than a two percent chance of becoming pregnant while experiencing amenorrhea during the first six months postpartum.[24,25] The high infertility noted *during*

Notes

---

[22] After six months postpartum, the baby receives other nourishment in addition to breast milk, and the mother is in the category of *continued breastfeeding.*

[23] K. Kennedy, R. Rivera, and A. McNeilly, "Consensus statement on the use of breastfeeding as a family planning method," *Contraception* 39:5 (May 1989) 477–496. From the Bellagio Consensus Conference on Lactational Infertility, Bellagio, Italy, August 1988.

[24] The *Consensus Statement* used the terms "Fully or nearly fully breastfeeding" and it was defined as exclusive breastfeeding or nearly exclusive with slight supplementation, from a few swallows up to less than one feeding per day. The Couple to Couple League uses the term "exclusive breastfeeding" because it is a commonly used medical term; however, CCL's definition is stronger as it allows no supplementation.

[25] A. Perez, M. Labbok, and J. Queenan, "A Clinical Study of the Lactational Amenorrhea Method for Family Planning," *Lancet* 339 (1992) 968–970.

the first six months (approximately 98%) for *exclusively breastfeeding mothers in amenorrhea* has been substantiated repeatedly in subsequent studies.[26,27,28,29] In fact, the evidence is so solid that it is classified as its own method of family planning (with its own set of guidelines) and is called the **Lactational Amenorrhea Method (LAM)**.[30]

Continued breastfeeding means nursing beyond six months, when other foods and liquids are added to complement the breast milk. The baby still nurses and pacifies at the breast on his own schedule. The increased duration of breastfeeding brings significant health and development benefits to the child and the mother. It can lead to extended infertility, beyond one year. During this time, a baby usually nurses less for nutrition and more for comfort. The AAP strongly encourages continued breastfeeding, even going so far as to state: "There is no upper limit to the duration of breastfeeding and no evidence of psychologic or developmental harm from breastfeeding into the third year of life or longer."[31]

Notes

[26] K. Kennedy, M. Labbok, and P. Van Look, "Consensus Statement: Lactational Amenorrhea Method for Family Planning," *Int J Gynaecol Obstet* 54 (1996) 55–57.

[27] World Health Organization Task Force on Methods for the Natural Regulation of Fertility, "The World Health Organization multinational study of breast-feeding and lactational amenorrhea. IV. Postpartum bleeding and lochia in breast-feeding women," *Fertil Steril* 72:3 (1999) 441–447.

[28] Ibid., 431–440.

[29] M. Labbok, V. Hight-Laukaran, Anne Peterson, Veronica Fletcher, Helena von Hertzen, Paul Van Look, et al., "Multicenter Study of the Lactational Amenorrhea Method (LAM) I. Efficacy, Duration, and Implications for Clinical Application," *Contraception* 55 (May/June 1997) 327–336.

[30] The Couple to Couple League does not promote exclusive breastfeeding as a method of family planning. This information is included because it has been well studied and has contributed significantly to our overall knowledge regarding the relationship between exclusive breastfeeding, amenorrhea, and infertility.

[31] 2005 AAP Policy Statement, 500.

Fertility Awareness after Childbirth

6

Lesson 6

Although most new birth mothers will experience at least a few weeks of postpartum amenorrhea, at some point in time most of you will return to your pre-pregnancy menstrual cycle lengths. How soon this occurs is highly dependent on the type of baby feeding you choose. This lesson will examine the key measurable signs of hormonal interactions — mucus, temperature, and cervix — as they occur during the postpartum transition, and explain how to interpret them, beginning with fertility awareness for formula feeding mothers. If you have given birth to other children, and you are using the same type of baby feeding with this infant, then you should also consider your past experience as you anticipate the return of fertility.

The graphic on the next page illustrates a typical transition for formula feeding mothers: from fertility cycles, to pregnancy and childbirth, followed by lochia, and a return to fertility cycles.

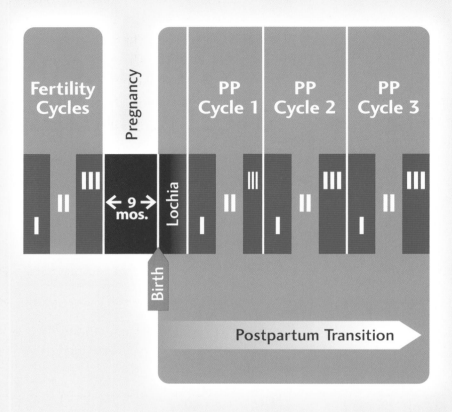

Note that you may initially experience a few overall longer cycles that have a longer Phase II and a shorter luteal phase before your cycles return to their pre-pregnancy lengths. A non-lactating mother generally experiences an early return of fertility because she is not producing lactating hormones to inhibit ovulation. Studies show that by the end of the third month postpartum, 91% of non-lactating mothers have had at least one period,[32] an indication that fertility is returning. Thus, couples need to know when to begin observing and charting the three key fertility signs in order to identify the return of fertility.

The three key fertility signs:

1. Mucus

While some formula feeding mothers may experience one or two **anovulatory cycles** (menstrual "cycles" without ovulation) prior to the first ovulation, others will not. Thus,

---

[32] Ruth Lawrence and Robert Lawrence, *Breastfeeding: A Guide for the Medical Professional* (Elsevier Mosby, 2005) 738.

it is important to begin making mucus observations and charting the mucus sign as soon as the lochia lessens. You can assume Phase I infertility, and, when you can resume marital relations according to your doctor's instructions, you should use the Phase I guidelines found on page 4 (limit marital relations to evenings of dry/nothing mucus days and abstain on any day that follows marital relations unless you are experienced and can positively detect the absence of mucus). When mucus sensations or characteristics return, you should assume Phase II fertility. (Note: If you are just learning NFP, CCL recommends that you abstain from genital contact for two weeks once the lochia lessens, and try to detect the absence or presence of any mucus sensations or characteristics. Record your observations on the chart and discuss with your CCL Teaching Couple or home study consultant after two weeks.)

The three key fertility signs:
2. Temperature

In addition to observing your mucus signs, begin taking your temperatures at three weeks postpartum.

Be sure to record both mucus and temperature signs on the chart, and apply the Sympto-Thermal Rule when possible.

The three key fertility signs:
3. Cervix

As you may recall from previous classes, the cervix observation is optional with regard to the Sympto-Thermal Method of NFP. After childbirth, it is important to note that the cervix needs time to heal and should not be examined until *your doctor gives permission to resume sexual intercourse with your husband.* If you are familiar with the cervix observation and this is your first baby, you will probably notice that the cervix seems more open than previously. In a sense, you may need to re-learn how the cervix feels when it is closed and open, and when it is hard and soft.

If you are unfamiliar with the cervix observation but would like to try it, you may find it helpful to check the cervix at the same time every day while you are learning,[33] in the afternoon and in the evening. For beginners, it is best to start the cervix check during Phase III because it is easier to locate the cervix at this time, and it will provide you with a baseline with which to compare the cervix checks you do in future cycles. In each cycle, begin

---

[33] Josef Roetzer, *Natural Conception Regulation (Natuerliche Empfaengnisregelung)* (Freiburg: Herder, 2006) 84.

checking the cervix as soon as menstruation decreases or by Cycle Day 6, whichever comes first. Be sure to follow the procedures explained in Class 1 (*The Art of Natural Family Planning® Student Guide*, pages 33–34 and 224).

Summary of Fertility Awareness When Formula Feeding

Everything that you have just learned with regard to applying fertility awareness while you are formula feeding can be summarized as follows:

- As soon as the lochia lessens, start mucus observations
  - Assume Phase I infertility and use the Phase I guidelines
  - When mucus signs and/or bleeding return, assume Phase II fertility
- Begin taking temperatures at three weeks
- Make the optional cervix exam *when you can resume marital relations as per your doctor's instructions*
- Chart fertility signs
- Apply the ST Rule when possible

Notes

The practice chart below illustrates how to interpret your fertility signs if you are feeding your baby formula.

Formula Feeding › Practice Chart

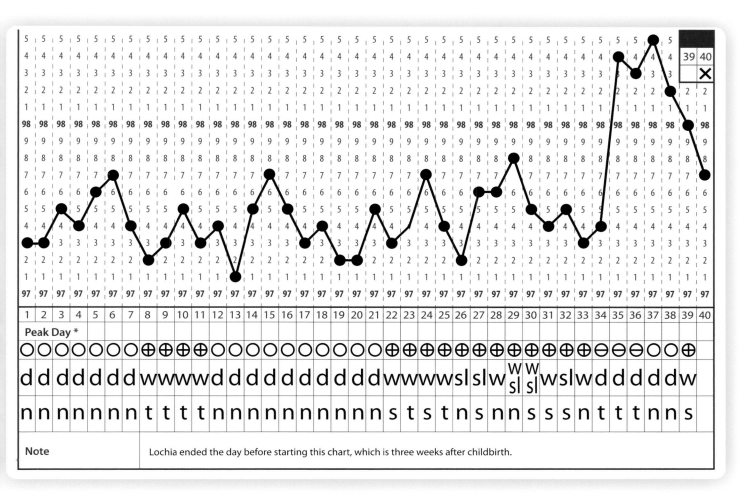

| Note | Lochia ended the day before starting this chart, which is three weeks after childbirth. |

If you are attending the Postpartum Class, you will complete this exercise in class. If you are using this Postpartum Student Guide on your own, be sure to check your answers on pages 56–57 of the Appendix.

1. Mark Peak Day and number the dry-up days that follow (e.g., P123).

2. Determine the preshift six temperatures.

3. Set the LTL and HTL.

4. Apply the ST Rule to determine the beginning of Phase III infertility. Draw a vertical line through the temperature and circle that cycle day on the chart.

Note that if you look at this chart one day at a time, mucus is detected on Cycle Days 8–11, followed by several days of no mucus sensations or characteristics. Look carefully at Cycle Day 11. Many might consider this to be Peak Day. However, because the mucus characteristics on Cycle Days 8–11 remain less-fertile (tacky) and do not progress to more-fertile (stretchy), and there is no thermal shift, the couple should still assume Phase II fertility. Peak Day actually occurs later in the cycle (Cycle Day 33) after the mother experiences a more substantial mucus build-up over several days with progression to more-fertile sensations and characteristics, followed by a dry-up and a thermal shift.

This chart also illustrates a Phase II that is longer than usual (note the delayed temperature rise that begins on Cycle Day 35) with a short luteal phase (in this case, five days). Both of these occurrences are typical for the first few cycles after childbirth. In addition, the temperature on Cycle Day 40 indicates a drop below the LTL and the beginning of a true menstruation.

Note that initially, you may experience cycles that are much longer than a normal pre-pregnancy cycle would be. In addition, you may have a longer than usual Phase II and a shorter than usual luteal phase. Such cycles are normal during the postpartum transition. The cycles will gradually shorten, while the luteal phases will gradually lengthen to your pre-pregnancy lengths. *The menstrual cycles that occur during this time of transition should not be considered or included when you are transferring data to a new chart each time a cycle begins.*

Breastfeeding

As you learned in the previous lesson, mothers who do not breastfeed generally have an earlier return of fertility than breastfeeding mothers. However, the delay of fertility in breastfeeding mothers can vary. It is much more significant for mothers who exclusively breastfeed their infants than it is for mothers who provide mixed breastfeeding. It is not uncommon to notice an absence of fertility signs for quite some time, especially if you are exclusively breastfeeding. When the signs of fertility do begin to appear, instead of immediately returning to menstrual cycles that pass through Phases I, II, and III, you may shift back and forth between Phase I and Phase II for a while before experiencing the first postpartum ovulation.

Husbands can be especially helpful during this time by encouraging their wives to get back into the routine of observing their fertility signs daily, and by recording this information for their wives on the chart.

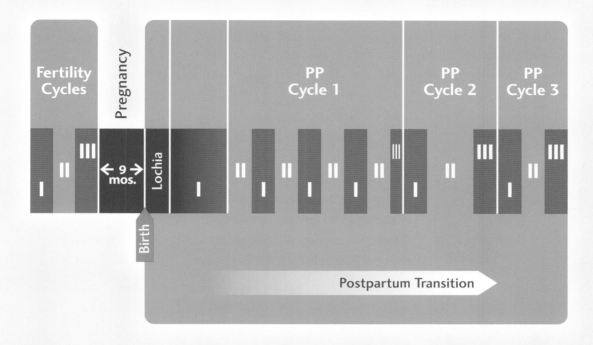

The graphic above illustrates this changing pattern for a nursing mother: from fertility cycles, to pregnancy and childbirth, followed by lochia and breastfeeding amenorrhea, and a return to fertility cycles. After the lochia dissipates, you will experience breastfeeding amenorrhea. This length of time depends on the many factors discussed in Lesson 5. Depending on those factors and your own physiology, your fertility will gradually return. It is common to experience a period of time characterized by a combination of days with fertility signs followed by days without fertility signs, as well as non-menstrual bleeding, before you have your first postpartum menstrual cycle. Usually, cycles return to their pre-pregnancy lengths after three cycles postpartum.

Earlier in this class, you reviewed the guidelines and rules that help you to know whether you are in Phase I, II, or III during a normal menstrual cycle. It is essential to understand this information in the context of the postpartum transition if you are breastfeeding.

The ST Rule is straightforward in determining the start of Phase III infertility and is used nearly every cycle by women during their fertile years. However, suckling increases prolactin, which suppresses LH, thereby delaying ovulation for a period of time. During this time, then, it is very important to understand and to follow guidelines to determine whether you are in Phase I infertility or Phase II fertility.

Postpartum Phase I and Phase II Guidelines for Marital Relations

Phase I

Evenings only of dry/nothing days: Remember that an infertile day is only determined after checking for mucus throughout the day. Therefore, you should start mucus observations as soon as the lochia lessens. You may not notice any mucus during the day, but then

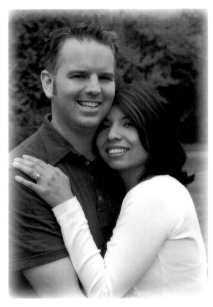

detect some mucus in the evening. If this occurs, consider yourself in Phase II because you detected mucus. (Note: If you are just learning NFP, CCL recommends that you abstain from genital contact for two weeks once the lochia lessens, and try to detect the absence or presence of any mucus sensations or characteristics. Record your observations on the chart and discuss with your NFP Teaching Couple or home study consultant after two weeks.)

Not on consecutive days: Marital relations usually leave seminal residue in the vaginal area. If you detect this residue during your mucus checks the following day, the seminal residue could mask the presence of mucus. You cannot assume you are infertile until you can positively assure yourself that there is no mucus present. Therefore, you should abstain on any day that follows marital relations in Phase I unless you are experienced and can positively detect dry sensations and no mucus characteristics.

Phase II

Assume Phase II fertility when:

- Mucus sensations or characteristics are detected
- Spotting or bleeding is not preceded by a thermal shift (possible breakthrough bleeding)

Be sure to take temperatures to establish the pre-shift six and LTL.

Notes

You will understand these guidelines better as you apply them in the context of the three key measurable signs of fertility.

The three key measurable signs of fertility:

1. Mucus

Mucus may vary during breastfeeding. It could be:
- Absent
- The same as pre-pregnancy
- In patches
- Present with spotting or bleeding
- Continuous

- ## When Mucus Is Absent

The absence of both mucus sensations and mucus characteristics indicates infertility. Thus, if you have no mucus, consider yourself in Phase I infertility.

- ## When Mucus Is the Same as During Pre-pregnancy Cycles

If the mucus signs are the same as during your pre-pregnancy cycles, follow the standard rules of mucus interpretation that you have already learned:

- Mucus sensations and/or characteristics indicate the start of Phase II fertility

- Find the Peak Day

- Apply the Sympto-Thermal Rule

These two conditions — when mucus is absent or the same as pre-pregnancy — are somewhat straightforward. However, it is not uncommon for breastfeeding mothers to encounter situations in which mucus sensations and characteristics appear and disappear as patches that come and go without a thermal shift occurring.

- ## When Mucus Appears in Patches

Mucus Patches *are defined as one or more days of mucus sensations/characteristics followed by dry/nothing days, without a thermal shift*. In such cases, any days with mucus sensations and/or mucus characteristics (less-fertile or more-fertile) are considered fertile.

To interpret a mucus patch, **mark the last day of the patch as Peak Day**. Note, however, that the term Peak Day used here carries a meaning unlike the one you learned previously in CCL's main NFP course. In the main course, you learned that Peak Day refers to the last day of the more-fertile mucus that occurs at ovulation, and is subsequently followed by a *drying-up process along with a thermal shift*. In the context in which it is presented here,

Peak Day refers to the last day of a mucus patch.

It is recorded the same, but interpreted differently in this particular situation because it is the last day of *any* mucus present (not just more-fertile mucus), and *there has been no ovulation, and thus, **no** thermal shift*. This means that no ST Rule is used and no Phase III is reached. Rather, when you have four days of dry sensations and no mucus characteristics after Peak Day (P1234), you return to Phase I infertility. This is called the **Mucus Patch Rule**.

 RULE *Mucus Patch Rule: Phase I infertility returns on the evening of the fourth day of no mucus sensations or characteristics after Peak Day, where Peak Day is the last day of a mucus patch or breakthrough bleeding.*[34]

It is important to note that if the temperatures begin to rise, the Mucus Patch Rule does not apply; wait for the start of Phase III according to the ST Rule.

Notes

---

[34] The Mucus Patch Rule application when breakthrough bleeding occurs is explained in the next section, "When Breakthrough Bleeding (Non-menstrual Spotting or Bleeding) Occurs," on pages 32–36.

The following practice chart illustrates how to interpret fertility signs when the mucus appears on and off in patches, without a thermal shift.

Patches of Mucus › Practice Chart

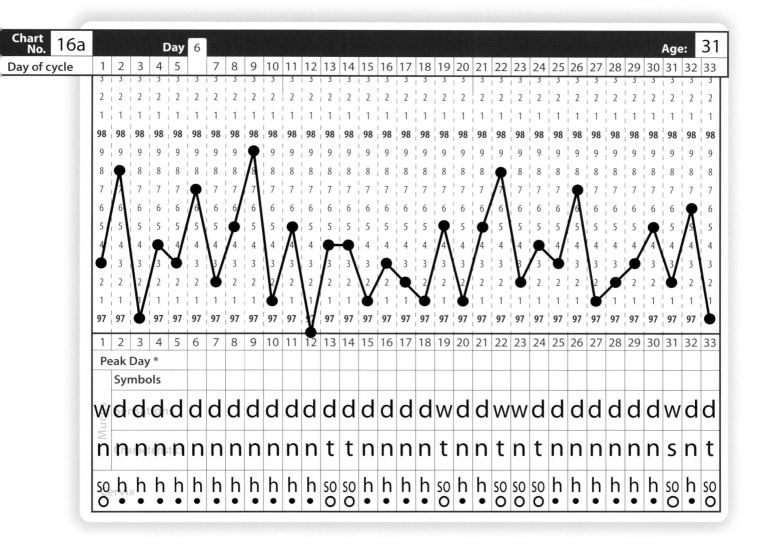

If you are attending the Postpartum Class, you will complete this exercise in class. If you are using this Postpartum Student Guide on your own, be sure to check your answers on page 58 of the Appendix.

1. For each cycle day, record the correct symbol.

2. Mark the Peak Day(s) and number the dry/nothing mucus days that follow (e.g., P1234).

3. The temperatures on this chart are up and down, with no indication of a thermal shift, and thus no Phase III. Because the mucus appears and disappears, and the fertility signs indicate that ovulation has not yet occurred, apply the Mucus Patch Rule where appropriate, and determine when this mother returns to Phase I infertility and when she enters Phase II fertility.

4. Draw a vertical phase division line between the last day of Phase I and the first day of Phase II. Indicate Phase I by writing the phase number "I" on the appropriate side of the vertical line, or mark a "1" on each cycle day.

5. Draw the phase division lines through the temperature when going from Phase II to Phase I (because Phase I returns in the evening of that day), and circle that day. Indicate Phase II by writing the phase number "II" on the appropriate side of the vertical line, or mark a "2" on each day.

- ## When Breakthrough Bleeding (Non-menstrual Spotting or Bleeding) Occurs

You will note that the Mucus Patch Rule includes situations in which a nursing mother may experience a bleeding episode that is not part of menstruation — days of spotting or bleeding that are not preceded by a thermal shift. This is called **breakthrough bleeding**. It can appear as spotting or bleeding in the middle of a cycle, and it can also appear as a regular menstrual flow following an anovulatory cycle. Breakthrough bleeding can mask the presence of mucus, making it a potentially fertile time, so you should follow the postpartum Phase II guidelines previously discussed in this lesson. If the bleeding is followed by days without mucus (dry sensations and no characteristics), then

Peak Day refers to the last day of the breakthrough bleeding.

As with mucus patches, when you have four days of dry sensations and no mucus characteristics after Peak Day (P1234), and there are no temperatures in a rising pattern, you return to Phase I infertility.

The next practice exercise illustrates how to determine the fertile and infertile days in this situation.

Notes

Breakthrough Bleeding › Practice 1

Chart No. 1		Day 6																													Age: 28	
Day of cycle	1	2	3	4	5		7	8	9	10	11	12	13	14	15	16	17	18	19	20	21	22	23	24	25	26	27	28	29	30	31	32	33
Menstruation	X	X	X	X	X	X	X	/																	/	/	/	/	/					

(temperature grid chart, rows 2,1,98,9,8,7,6,5,4,3,2,1,97 with connected temperature dots across days 1–33)

| 1 | 2 | 3 | 4 | 5 | 6 | 7 | 8 | 9 | 10 | 11 | 12 | 13 | 14 | 15 | 16 | 17 | 18 | 19 | 20 | 21 | 22 | 23 | 24 | 25 | 26 | 27 | 28 | 29 | 30 | 31 | 32 | 33 |

Peak Day *

Mucus																																		
Symbols				O	O	O	O	O	O	O	O	O	O	O	O	O	O	O	O	O	⊕	⊖	⊖	⊖	⊖	⊖	O	O	O	O	O		
Sensations (couldn't assess)				d	d	d	d	d	d	d	d	d	d	d	d	d	d	d	w	couldn't assess sensation						d	d	d	d	d		
Characteristics (couldn't assess)				n	n	n	n	n	n	n	n	n	n	n	n	n	n	n	n	t	t	t	t	t	n	n	n	n	n		

Note	Began charting when bleeding appeared; no mucus prior to that.

If you are attending the Postpartum Class, you will complete this exercise in class. If you are using this Postpartum Student Guide on your own, be sure to check your answers on pages 59–60 of the Appendix.

1. Mark the Peak Day and number the dry/nothing mucus days that follow (e.g., P1234).

2. Apply the Mucus Patch Rule to determine the return to Phase I infertility.

3. Draw a vertical phase division line between the last day of Phase I and the first day of Phase II. Indicate Phase I by writing the phase number "I" on the appropriate side of the vertical line, or mark a "1" on each day.

4. Draw the phase division lines through the temperature when going from Phase II to Phase I and circle that day. Indicate Phase II by writing the phase number "II" on the appropriate side of the vertical line, or by marking a "2" for each day.

When Mucus Follows Breakthrough Bleeding

Physiologically, breakthrough bleeding usually occurs when the endometrium builds up so much that the top layer cannot be sustained solely by estrogen, so the endometrium breaks down, and spotting or bleeding results. It is important to be aware that mucus may be present during and/or immediately after this bleeding episode. Thus, if the bleeding is followed by days with mucus sensations and/or characteristics, then

> **Peak Day refers to the last day of the mucus patch that follows the breakthrough bleeding.**

As in the preceding examples of mucus patches and breakthrough bleeding, when you have four days of dry sensations and no mucus characteristics after Peak Day (P1234), and there are no temperatures in a rising pattern, you return to Phase I infertility. Apply the **Mucus Patch Rule** as follows:

> **Phase I infertility returns on the evening of the fourth day of no mucus sensations or characteristics after Peak Day, where Peak Day is the last day of a mucus patch or breakthrough bleeding.**

The next practice exercise illustrates how to determine the fertile and infertile days when this situation occurs.

Notes

Chart No.	1 after childbirth																														Age:	26
Day of cycle	1	2	3	4	5	6	7	8	9	10	11	12	13	14	15	16	17	18	19	20	21	22	23	24	25	26	27	28	29	30	31	32	33
Menstruation														/	X	X	X	/	/	•													

Temperature grid scale (repeated each column): 2, 1, 98, 9, 8, 7, 6, 5, 4, 3, 2, 1, 97

	1	2	3	4	5	6	7	8	9	10	11	12	13	14	15	16	17	18	19	20	21	22	23	24	25	26	27	28	29	30	31	32	33

Peak Day *

Mucus characteristics																																	
⊕	⊕	⊕	⊕	⊕	⊕	⊕	⊕	⊕	⊕	⊕	⊕							⊕	⊕	⊖	○	○	○	○	○	○	○	○	○	⊖	⊖	⊕	○
w	w	w	w	w	w	w	w	w	w	w	w	w	blood	blood	blood	blood	blood	blood	w	w	d	d	d	d	d	d	d	d	d	d	w	d
s	s	s	s	s	s	s	s	s	s	s	s	s							t	n	t	n	n	n	n	n	n	n	t	t	n		

Note	Began charting when fertility signs first appeared.

If you are attending the Postpartum Class, you will complete this exercise in class. If you are using this Postpartum Student Guide on your own, be sure to check your answers on page 61 of the Appendix.

1. Mark the Peak Day(s) and number the dry/nothing mucus days that follow (e.g., P1234).

2. Apply the Mucus Patch Rule to determine the return to Phase I infertility.

3. Draw a vertical phase division line between the last day of Phase I and the first day of Phase II. Indicate Phase I by writing the phase number "I" on the appropriate side of the vertical line, or mark a "1" on each day.

4. Draw the phase division lines through the temperature when going from Phase II to Phase I and circle that day. Indicate Phase II by writing the phase number "II" on the appropriate side of the vertical line, or by marking a "2" for each day.

This chart illustrates a combination of breakthrough bleeding and mucus patches. The last day of the spotting/bleeding that occurs on Cycle Days 14–20 is also the first day of a three-day patch of mucus (wet/tacky, wet/nothing, and dry/tacky). Another patch of mucus begins on Cycle Day 30.

- Continuous Mucus

The postpartum transition is quite unique, and as you have seen from the previous examples, it differs from regular cycles because you may experience patches of mucus and even breakthrough bleeding without ovulation. In addition to these more common experiences, a postpartum woman may notice **continuous mucus**, a mucus pattern that seems different from the variations previously discussed. Continuous mucus may manifest itself in two ways.

One type of continuous mucus could be an **unchanging mucus pattern**. *Unchanging* means that *the mucus sensations, characteristics, and quantity remain the same; they do not change.* An unchanging mucus pattern might appear right after the lochia ends or later, and may remain, sometimes for a period of time. If you should notice this, be sure to record your observations on your chart, along with a brief written description of the sensations and/or characteristics in the notes section or on a separate piece of paper. (See example below.) While you are observing and recording this mucus, abstain from genital contact and begin taking your temperature. If the unchanging mucus pattern continues for two weeks, **talk to your CCL Teaching Couple**, or if you are taking the Home Study Course, contact your consultant, who is listed in the "How to Get Started" insert located in your home study kit. (For more information, see the Reference Guide, page 64.)

41	42	43	44	45	46	47	48	49	50	51	52	53	54	55	56	57	58	59	60	61	62
Peak Day *																					
Symbols																					
d	d	d	d	d	d	d	d	d	d	d	d	d	d	d	d	d	d	d	d	d	d
t	t	t	t	t	t	t	t	t	t	t	t	t	t	t	t	t	t	t	t	t	t
Note	Dry sensation and little clumps of white mucus every day																				

A second type of continuous mucus that could occur in the postpartum transition is one that consists of a **changing mucus pattern**. What is meant by *a changing mucus pattern* is that *the mucus sensations and/or characteristics change frequently, but do not disappear* as they would if the woman was having mucus patches. In a changing mucus pattern a woman may notice an occasional dry/nothing mucus day, but not four or more days with dry sensations and no mucus characteristics. For the postpartum woman who is breastfeeding, the more common time to experience a changing mucus pattern is when the baby is several months old and receiving complementary foods, etc. This is a distinctive time for a mother because, on the one hand, her ovaries are preparing for an ovulation since sufficient time has passed after childbirth; yet, on the other hand, the baby is nursing frequently enough to prevent the ovaries from completely ripening a follicle for ovulation to occur. The end result is that mucus is observed almost daily, which can alternate from more- to less-fertile or vice versa. Basically, there is an internal *tug-of-war* occurring between the woman's ovaries that are trying to mature a follicle for ovulation, and her pituitary gland that is producing scarcely enough prolactin to suppress the complete development of the ovarian follicle. That is why she may observe this relatively long period of a changing mucus pattern (e.g. six to eight weeks).

Understanding that this *tug-of-war* phenomenon is a normal development for many women as ovulation or the return of the menstrual cycles approaches can alleviate undue concern, especially when a couple desires to postpone a pregnancy at the present time.

Notes

Should you experience a changing mucus pattern, assume you are in Phase II, and follow the ST Rule and guidelines if you are avoiding a pregnancy.

Note the example of a changing mucus pattern below.

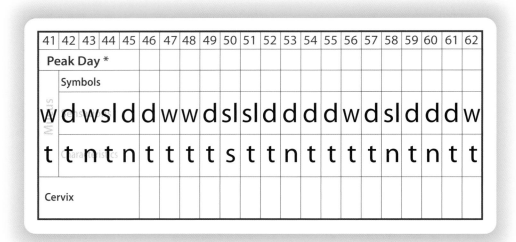

Note that not all discharges are cervical mucus, and some could be the result of an infection. Infections are characterized generally by an odor and/or unusual type of discharge, which could be irritating or painful. If you experience such a discharge, contact your doctor for an evaluation. (See the Reference Guide, *Vaginal Discharges,* in *The Art of Natural Family Planning® Student Guide,* pages 268–269.)

The three key measurable signs of fertility:

2. Temperature

During a normal fertile cycle, after ovulation the empty egg follicle becomes a structure called the corpus luteum, and it begins to produce progesterone. The progesterone causes your basal body temperature to rise, which begins the **luteal phase** — the number of days between the first day of temperature rise and the next menstruation. Breastfeeding mothers may experience a long period of time with no ovulations. If there is no ovulation, then there will also be no corpus luteum and no progesterone. Without progesterone, there will be no temperature rise.

Therefore, breastfeeding mothers do not need to record their temperature sign until they detect mucus sensations, mucus characteristics, spotting, or bleeding. If you are breastfeeding, you should start recording your temperatures as soon as you experience any of these symptoms of fertility. Once a thermal shift occurs, apply the ST Rule. (Note that normally your temperatures will not be affected by the routine care of your baby during the night. However, you should note on your chart any unusual nighttime disturbances, such as being up for several hours with a sick baby.)

The three key measurable signs of fertility:
3. Cervix

As you learned in Class 1, the cervix indicates fertility when it is open and/or soft; it indicates infertility when it is both closed and hard.

Although this sign is optional, it can be particularly helpful for breastfeeding mothers during the postpartum transition. It can confirm the other key signs of fertility, and sometimes it can eliminate confusion when these signs are difficult to interpret. For example, occasionally you may have missed temperature readings if you had a difficult night, or the temperatures may be abnormal due to illness or other stressful situations. In such cases, women who have experience using the cervix sign may find it especially helpful in determining days of fertility and infertility when it is used along with the mucus sign.

Just as with the mucus sign, the cervix may change from indicating infertility earlier in the day to signifying fertility several hours later. Remember that you are looking for a *change* in the cervix: from closed and hard to open and soft.

The following recommendations summarize how to use the cervix sign most effectively during the postpartum transition when you are breastfeeding.

Resume the cervix exam

- When you can resume marital relations *as per your doctor's instructions* **AND**
- When other observations indicate that fertility could be returning

Make cervix observations

- At the same time each day
- Afternoon and evening
- Follow procedures explained in Class 1

If you are making the cervix observation, be sure to record this sign on the chart along with your mucus and temperature signs. Apply the ST Rule when possible. The chart on the next page illustrates how the cervix sign corresponds with the mucus signs as one woman's fertility is returning after childbirth.

Chart No.	12																										Age:	29
Day of cycle	34	35	36	37	38	39	40	41	42	43	44	45	46	47	48	49	50	51	52	53	54	55	56	57	58	59	60
Menstruation						•	•	•	•	•	•	•														/	

Note that this chart only includes the data for Cycle Days 34–59. The "P" on Cycle Day 34 indicates the last day of a mucus patch, but after three dry/nothing days, there is another day of mucus, followed by several days of a bloody discharge, more mucus that becomes more-fertile, and finally, ovulation. The open and soft cervix signs confirmed that the days of bloody discharge were indications that fertility was returning. These were followed by days of greatest fertility on Cycle Days 47–53 as evidenced by both the mucus and cervix signs. When the mucus became more-fertile and was followed by drying-up and a thermal shift (indicating that ovulation had occurred), the cervix sign along with the other signs of fertility confirmed that Phase III had begun. In this example, the cervix sign confirmed the start of Phase III a day earlier than if this sign had not been used.

Summary of Fertility Awareness When Breastfeeding

Everything that you have just learned with regard to applying fertility awareness while you are breastfeeding can be summarized as follows:

- As soon as the lochia lessens, start mucus observations
- When mucus signs and/or bleeding return
  - Assume Phase II fertility
  - Apply the Mucus Patch Rule if necessary
  - Begin taking temperatures
  - Make the optional cervix exam *when you can resume marital relations as per your doctor's instructions*
  - Chart fertility signs and record the type of breastfeeding in the Notes section of your chart
- Apply the ST Rule when possible

Note that initially, you may experience cycles that are much longer than a normal pre-pregnancy cycle would be. In addition, you may have longer than usual Phase II's and shorter than usual luteal phases. Such cycles are normal during the postpartum transition. The cycles will gradually shorten, while the luteal phases will gradually lengthen to your pre-pregnancy lengths. *The menstrual cycles that occur during this time of transition should not be considered or included when you are transferring data in the Cycle History box to a new chart each time a cycle begins. Use only your pre-pregnancy cycle history to calculate and apply Phase I rules.*

The next five charts demonstrate the return of fertility after childbirth for a mother who has been following the principles of exclusive and continued breastfeeding. As you learned in Class 2, it is important to complete the information on the chart concerning your previous cycle history. *Use information from your pre-pregnancy cycles.*

Notes

Exclusive Breastfeeding › No Ovulation

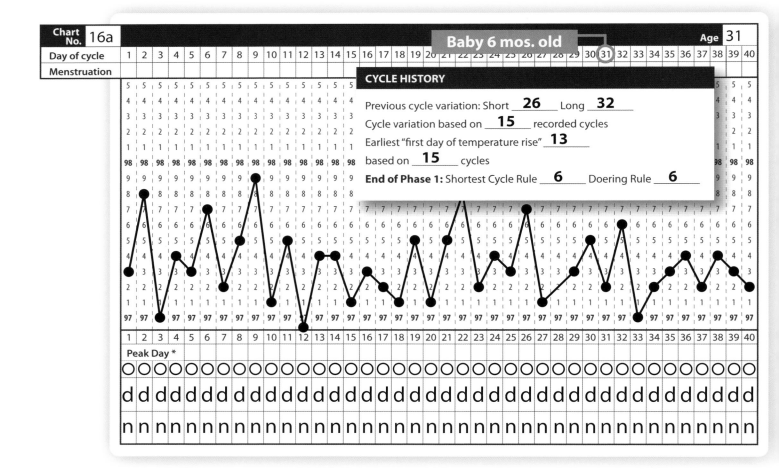

The first chart in this series is actually the sixteenth cycle (Chart No. 16a) for this woman, indicating that she is experienced in making and recording her fertility observations.

Even though this mother had not been observing any signs of fertility, she started charting in anticipation of the sixth month postpartum to see what her temperature and mucus signs would look like one month prior to the introduction of solids for her child. As you can see, there are no signs of fertility and no rising temperatures to indicate a thermal shift.

Continued Breastfeeding › No Ovulation

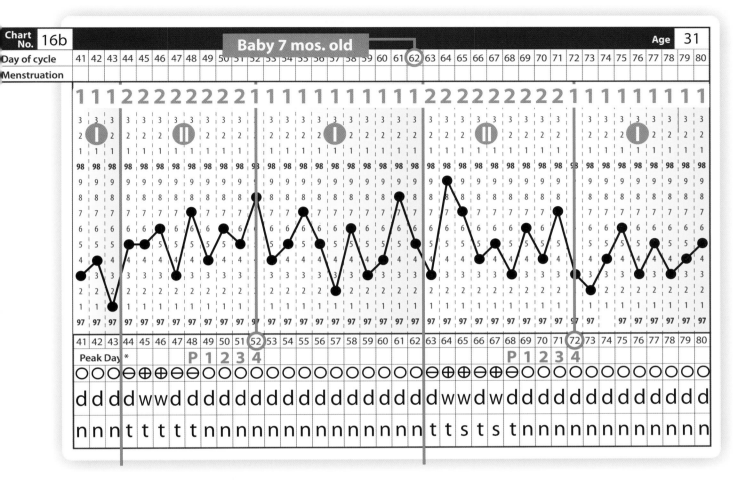

Chart No. 16b continues this same pattern with the appearance of some mucus on Cycle Days 44–48 and again on Cycle Days 63–68. On these days, the woman assumes fertility. However, the Mucus Patch Rule indicates the return to Phase I infertility on Cycle Days 52 and 72, respectively. Notice that there is no indication of a thermal shift.

Notes

Continued Breastfeeding › First Ovulation

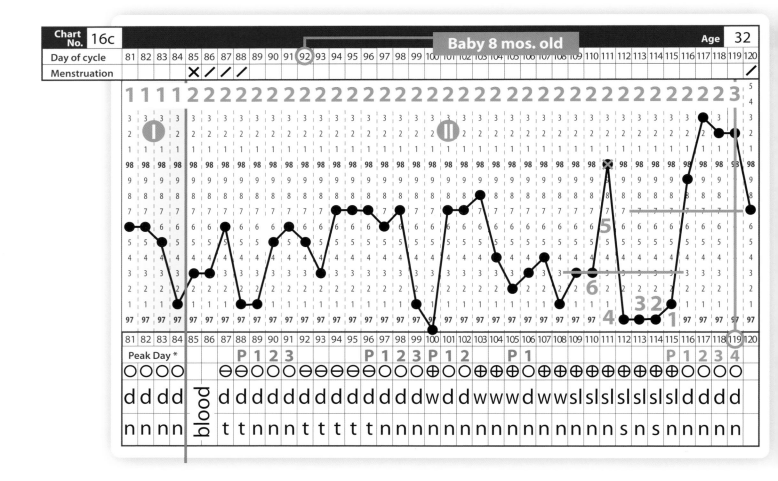

Chart No. 16c indicates breakthrough bleeding on Cycle Days 85–88. This chart illustrates more frequent patches of mucus, culminating with a thermal shift beginning on Cycle Day 116, and a very short luteal phase (four days). Menstruation begins on Cycle Day 120. This is the first postpartum ovulation for this mother. Subsequent ovulations can be expected as her fertility signs return to their pre-pregnancy patterns.

Notes

Continued Breastfeeding › Second Ovulation

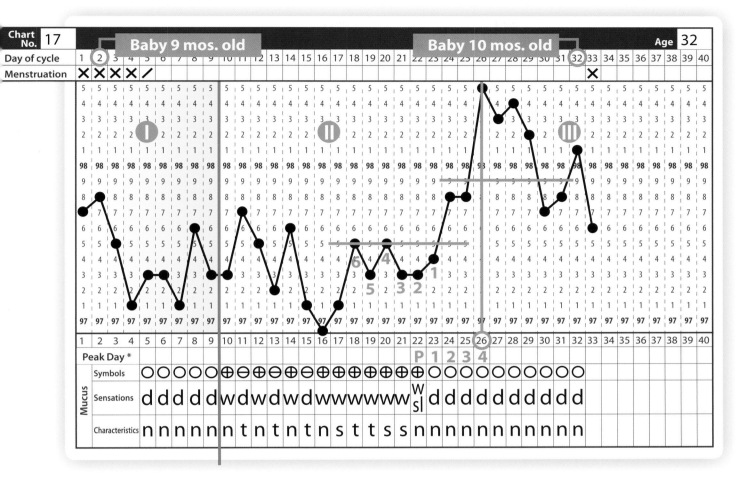

Chart No. 17 indicates the second ovulation postpartum and a longer luteal phase (nine days) than in the previous cycle.

Notes

Continued Breastfeeding › Third Ovulation

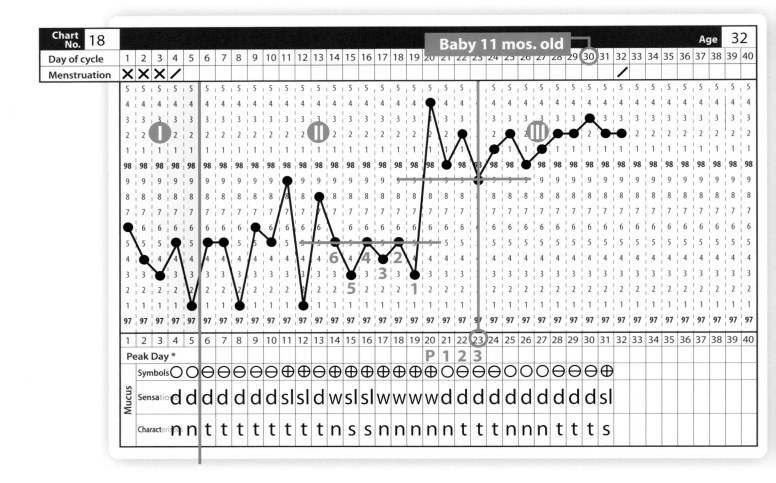

On Chart No. 18, you can see that she is still experiencing a slightly longer than usual Phase II fertility compared to a normal pre-pregnancy cycle, and that her luteal phase has increased three days (12 days) since the previous cycle.

These charts illustrate the delay in fertility that is a common experience for mothers who breastfeed their infants exclusively for six months, and add only complementary foods after that time.

Postpartum Decisions: NFP and Responsible Parenthood

7

Lesson 7

As you cradle your new baby in your arms and begin adjusting to your new roles as mom and dad, thoughts about welcoming the next child may be the farthest thing from your mind. It is good to remember, however, that the call to practice responsible parenthood is an ongoing one. Just as during times of normal fertility a couple is called to discern each month their readiness to seek or hope for a new life, the later months of pregnancy and the early postpartum weeks are indeed appropriate times for discussions and discernment about the timing of welcoming more children. During these earlier weeks, it is not unusual to feel overwhelmed at the thought of another child, but, with time, healing, and recovery these feelings can change. In reality, a woman's fertility may be many months — possibly even a year or more — away from returning (depending largely on the type of baby feeding that is chosen), but any couple could experience an earlier-than-expected return of fertility. Therefore, ongoing prayers and discussions about family size are important and will empower and prepare you no matter when fertility returns — even if that happens while you are still in the throes of adjusting to the little one in your arms now.

The Postpartum Time and Responsible Parenthood

The birth of a baby rightly brings much change in a family's routine as the need to care for this newest family member becomes paramount. Husbands are learning to be fathers, wives are learning to be mothers, and both are learning to relate to each other in new ways and with new perspectives of each other. And, if this baby is not the first, siblings are experiencing their own share of adjustment. Add to this the practical considerations of starting a family, possibly adjusting down to one income, moving to more appropriate housing, etc., and it is easy to see the importance of being open with each other, praying together, and hopefully being in agreement about your responsible parenthood decisions at this time.

Recall that responsible parenthood is the virtuous decision to plan or to postpone another child. Responsible parenthood involves basing your family size decisions in love — love for God, love for your spouse, and love for the children you already have. The Catholic

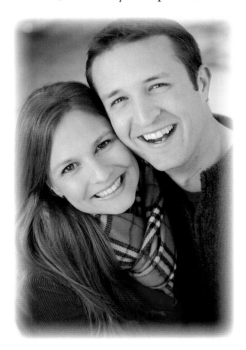

Church calls us to be generous by reminding us that children are the supreme gift of marriage. While the Church has provided broad guidance regarding just reasons for responsibly postponing conception in *Humanae Vitae*, and speaks of "physical, economic, psychological, and social" conditions,[35] it does not define these conditions. Thus, it is up to each married couple to prayerfully discern whether the conditions in their marriage and family are appropriate or not for trying to conceive another child at any given time.

The time of postpartum infertility that most women experience with exclusive and continued breastfeeding usually allows ample opportunity for discernment as parents. When your fertility returns, are you both ready to welcome another child at that time? Are the two of you physically, financially, and psychologically meeting the needs of the children you currently have? Would it be prudent to postpone a pregnancy because one or more of your children requires additional attention that really should come from you? Does mom need more time to recover from a physically demanding pregnancy? These are just a few examples of situations that may need to be carefully considered as you make future decisions regarding family size. Many couples have found that these responsible parenthood decisions are made easier through exclusive and continued breastfeeding with its usual duration of delayed ovulation and extended infertility. This allows the baby to be nurtured on his/her timetable, while mother and father experience a natural spacing between children.

Regardless of the form of baby feeding, if you experience the return of fertility signs and your prayerful discernment calls you to postpone the next pregnancy, NFP (fertility awareness) is still practiced by the observation of the signs (or lack of signs) of fertility and taking the necessary steps to abstain or not during the fertile days, depending upon your circumstances. As the postpartum months continue, perhaps you find that a situation that

---

35 Pope Paul VI, *On Human Life*, no. 10.

initially caused you to rely on fertility awareness in order to delay a pregnancy, changes after several more months of breastfeeding. Perhaps now you could be more open to another child. The beauty of NFP, even in the postpartum time, is that parents can change their minds from one "cycle" to another — from one day to another.

Balance is a key factor here as parents discern the needs of everyone in the family. Responsible parenthood is the virtuous and prudent decision to hope for another child, or to postpone or avoid conception for the good of the family. When a couple needs to postpone and they are beyond any natural infertility following childbirth, they can use their knowledge of fertility awareness to delay conception. This requires open and honest spousal communication, an art that is acquired through healthy marital intimacy.

Marital Intimacy

Intimacy involves the most private part of our being. **Marital intimacy** is much more than sexual intercourse; it involves both verbal and non-verbal communication about topics that are important to both spouses. This is especially important to keep in mind during these months of adjusting to new parenthood, which brings with it changes in the sexual relationship. In the midst of the excitement that surrounds the arrival of a new baby, it is also very important for you to set aside time to think, converse, pray, and just be together as husband and wife. It is not unusual for spouses to hit a few "bumps in the road" as they try to re-establish sexual intimacy following the birth of a new baby. Exhaustion, adjusting to new roles, the effects of breastfeeding hormones, fear of another pregnancy…many such factors can influence a couple's sexual intimacy. But when we strive to keep our priorities in order — God, spouse, family, others — then we can be better lovers and better parents.

Perhaps this is best expressed in the words of author C. S. Lewis in *Letters of C. S. Lewis* (November 1952): "When I have learnt to love God better than my earthly dearest, I shall love my earthly dearest better than I do now. In so far as I learn to love my earthly dearest at the expense of God and instead of God, I shall be moving toward the state in which I shall not love my earthly dearest at all. When first things are put first, second things are not suppressed but increased."

Notes

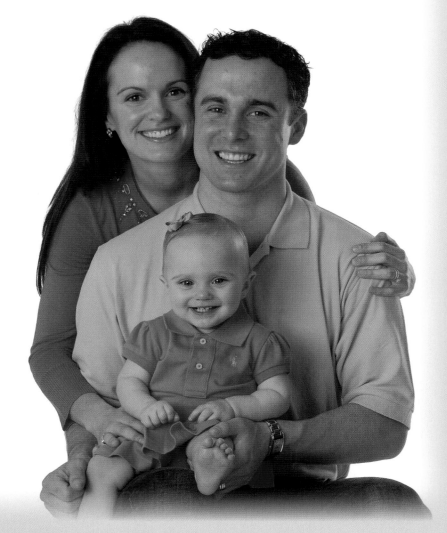

Next Steps

Now that you have completed the Postpartum Class, the next step is to complete the NFP course and apply what you have learned.

The Couple to Couple League invites you to call or email for assistance when necessary. It is best to contact a local certified CCL Teaching Couple. However, if this is not possible, you may contact the main office directly. NFP consulting is free for those who have received instruction from CCL (class series or Home Study Course) **and** have a current CCL membership. Others may receive consulting help for a fee.

In addition, as a member of the Couple to Couple League, you will find *Family Foundations* to be a regular useful resource for topics related to your fertility and breastfeeding. The CCL website, ***www.ccli.org***, contains additional information on this subject.

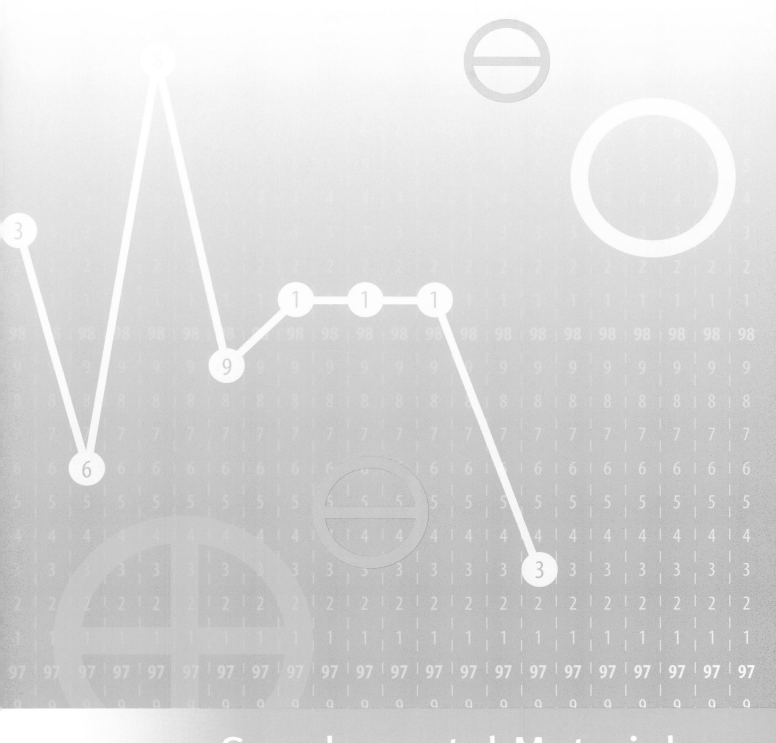

Supplemental Material

Appendix: Answers to Practice Charts

Practice Exercises	Pages

Steps for Applying the Sympto-Thermal Rule

1. Find the Peak Day and number the three days of drying up after it from left to right.

2. Find three temperatures higher than six preceding temperatures. (Remember, the three rising temperatures should be in close proximity to Peak Day.)

3. Number the pre-shift six from right to left.

4. Draw the Low Temperature Level (LTL) on the highest of the pre-shift six temperatures.

5. Draw the High Temperature Level (HTL) at 0.4° F above the LTL.

6. Find three normal post-peak temperatures. If all three temperatures are above the LTL, and the third temperature is at or above the HTL, Phase III begins on the evening of that day.

7. Check the cervix signs if recorded. If there are 3 days of a closed and hard cervix, then it is not necessary for the third normal post-peak temperature to reach the HTL. Phase III begins on the evening of that day.

8. If the requirements in steps #6 or #7 are not met, wait for an additional post-peak temperature above the LTL; Phase III begins on the evening of that day.

9. After you apply the ST Rule and determine the start of Phase III, draw a vertical phase division line through the temperature dot on the first day of Phase III.

Notes

Review › Practice Chart (page 6)

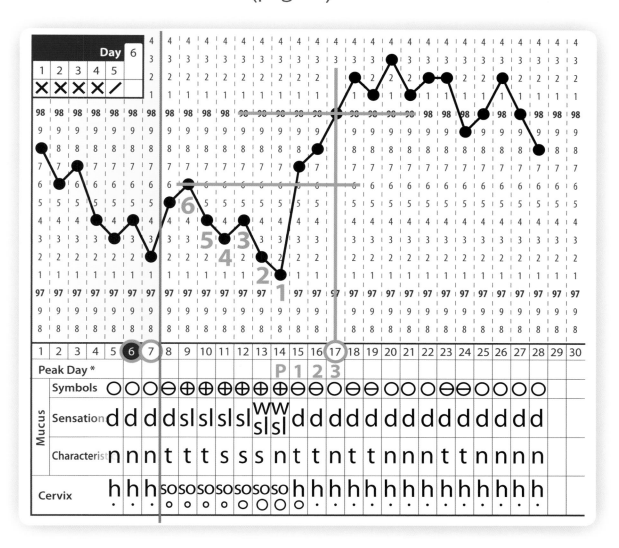

Phase I and Phase II:

- Shortest-Cycle Rule = Cycle Day 6

- Doering Rule = Cycle Day 7

- Last Dry Day Rule = Cycle Day 7

- End of Phase I = Cycle Day 7

Phase III:

Phase III begins on the evening of the third day of drying-up past the Peak Day combined with three normal post-peak temperatures (Cycle Day 14, plus Cycle Days 15, 16, 17), and the third temperature past the Peak Day is at or above the High Temperature Level (HTL) (yes). Since these conditions are met, there is no need to wait for three days with a closed and hard cervix or for an additional post-peak day for another temperature. Phase III begins on the evening of Cycle Day 17.

Formula Feeding › Practice Chart (page 25)

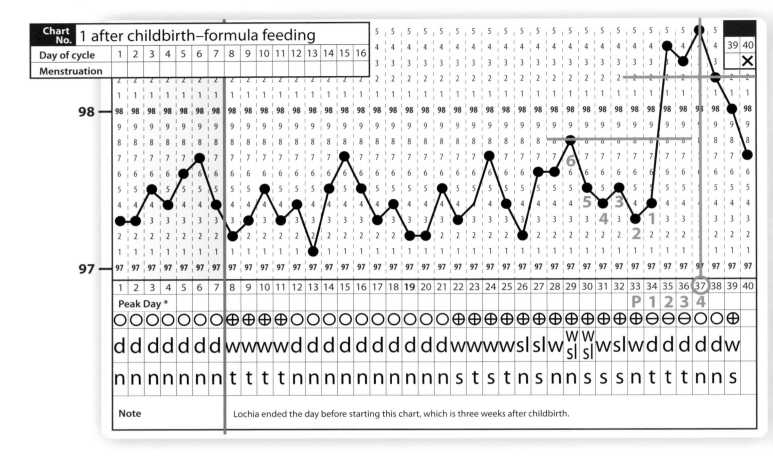

Phase I and Phase II:

- Shortest-Cycle Rule = Unknown
- Doering Rule = Unknown
- Last Dry Day Rule = Cycle Day 7
- End of Phase I = Cycle Day 7

Note: This first postpartum cycle has a very long Phase II, which is not unusual for the first full cycle after childbirth. Because this mother detected the beginning of mucus sensations and characteristics on Cycle Day 8, she knew she was in Phase II. Even though Cycle Days 12–21 indicated dry mucus sensations/no mucus characteristics, the mother continued her observations in anticipation of experiencing the more-fertile mucus signs (stretchy) in addition to the less-fertile (tacky). These signs appeared beginning on Cycle Day 22.

Phase III:

Phase III begins on the evening of the third day of drying-up past the Peak Day combined with three normal post-peak temperatures (Cycle Days 35, 36, 37), and the third temperature past the Peak Day is at or above the High Temperature Level (HTL) (yes). Since these conditions are met, Phase III begins on the evening of Cycle Day 37.

This chart illustrates the return of fertility for a mother who feeds her baby with a bottle.

Notes

Patches of Mucus › Practice Chart (page 31)

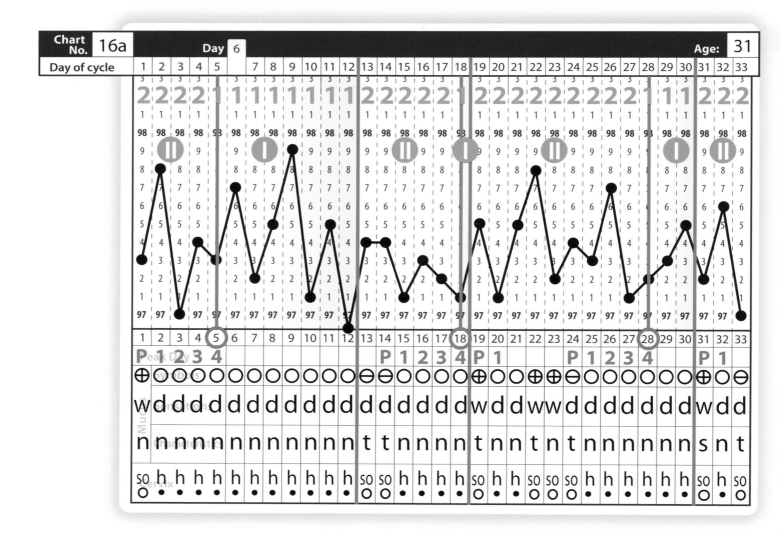

Phase II begins:

- Cycle Days 1, 13, 19, and 31

Phase I returns:

- Cycle Days 5, 18, and 28. Phase I infertility returns on the evening of the fourth day of no mucus sensations or characteristics after Peak Day (Cycle Days 5, 18, and 28), where Peak Day is the last day of a mucus patch or breakthrough bleeding (Cycle Days 1, 14, 19, 24, and 31).

Breakthrough Bleeding › Practice 1 (page 33)

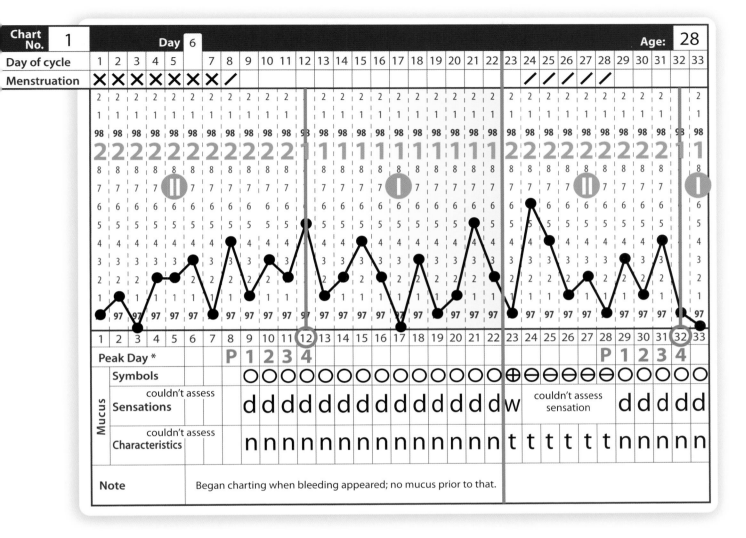

Phase II begins:

- Cycle Days 1 and 23

Phase I returns:

- Cycle Days 12 and 32. Phase I infertility returns on the evening of the fourth day of no mucus sensations or characteristics after Peak Day (Cycle Days 12 and 32), where Peak Day is the last day of a mucus patch or breakthrough bleeding (Cycle Days 8 and 28).

Note: The bleeding on Cycle Days 1–8 and 24–28 is not menstrual bleeding, but rather, breakthrough bleeding. These days are considered to be a potentially fertile time. Cycle Days 8 and 28 should be marked as Peak Days. The Patch Rule can be applied because the days that follow, Cycle Days 9–12 and 29–32, are four dry/nothing days and there is no thermal shift. These days should be numbered accordingly (e.g., 1234).

This chart illustrates what a breastfeeding mother may experience before she has her first postpartum ovulation.

Notes

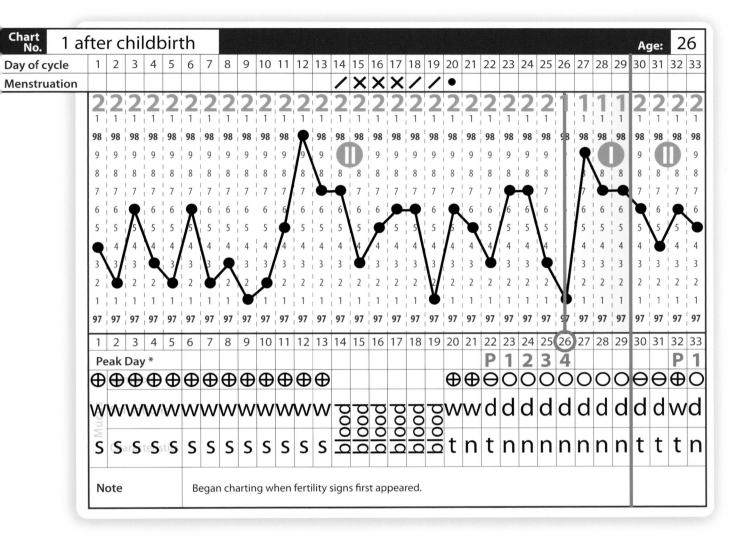

Phase II begins:

- Cycle Days 1 and 30

Phase I returns:

> Cycle Day 26. Phase I infertility returns on the evening of the fourth day of no mucus sensations or characteristics after Peak Day (Cycle Day 26), where Peak Day is the last day of a mucus patch or breakthrough bleeding (Cycle Days 22 and 32).

Note: In accordance with the Mucus Patch Rule, Peak Day is marked on Cycle Day 22 because it is the last day of the mucus patch that follows the breakthrough bleeding and there is no thermal shift.

R Reference Guide

Additional Resources

For more information on breastfeeding:

See *The Art of Breastfeeding* by Linda Kracht and Jackie Hilgert (The Couple to Couple League).

For thyroid-related problems:

If you notice many months of unusually low basal temperatures or if your cycles do not return to their pre-pregnancy lengths within a reasonable amount of time, you may find helpful information at: **www.brodabarnes.org**

To locate NFP-supportive physicians:

There are some physicians who do not prescribe or recommend contraception, sterilization or abortion; nor will some of them refer to another physician for these services. Instead, these NFP-supportive physicians use treatments that address a woman's underlying condition rather than trying to mask or further complicate them by prescribing hormones as a method of birth control. Such physicians are hard to find.

If you are interested in finding an NFP-supportive physician in your area, visit One More Soul's website at **www.omsoul.org**. One More Soul maintains a database of NFP-supportive physicians, which they term *NFP-Only,* and is the best source for this information.

In addition to the above, there are many physicians who are supportive of NFP, but who also prescribe hormones as a method of birth control. Often, such physicians can read an NFP chart and provide sound counsel to women. If you cannot find an NFP-Only physician in your area, seek one who supports NFP. There are many instances in which these physicians eventually discontinued prescribing or recommending birth control, sterilization or abortion after seeing many patients who understand their fertility signs and apply NFP. Prayer and subtle encouragement are common actions that can lead to conversion.

If you would like your physician or a physician in your area to learn what it means to maintain an NFP-supportive practice, CCL sponsors a Physician Seminar once each year. The CCL Physician Seminar is a great way to help your doctor, nurse, or health care professional better serve you and others in your area. The seminar consists of what couples learn in a CCL class — the Sympto-Thermal Method of NFP — and how couples chart using this method. These physicians are then better able to counsel women who have attended a CCL class since they are familiar with this method. The seminar also covers information about the return of fertility after childbirth and premenopause. Lastly, physicians hear success stories from other medical professionals who do not prescribe or recommend birth control, sterilization or abortion, and learn how to apply those principles in their own practices.

A CCL Physician Seminar is also fully accredited by the American Academy of Family Physicians, and physicians who attend receive credits for their annual Continuing Medical Education (CME) requirements. For more information on CCL's Physician Seminar or to download a brochure, visit CCL's website at *www.ccli.org/seminars*.

For information on clinical nutritionists:

Contact the International & American Associations of Clinical Nutritionists to locate a clinical nutritionist near you: *www.iaacn.org* or 972-407-9089

Nutrition and fertility information::

See *Fertility, Cycles & Nutrition* by Marilyn Shannon (The Couple to Couple League, 2009).

Nutritional response testing:

When faced with cycle irregularities such as an extended time of short luteal phases once your postpartum cycles have returned, it may be helpful to investigate what nutrients your body may be lacking. Nutritional response testing is a non-invasive, reasonably priced way to determine what specific nutrients the body needs to perform optimally. To find a licensed health care professional trained in this technique/therapy in your area, call Ulan Nutritional Systems, Inc. at 727-466-6069, Ext.306.

Continuous mucus — an unchanging pattern of mucus

During the postpartum transition, one cycle variation that can occur is continuous mucus that is unchanging.

Unchanging means that the mucus remains the same; it does not change. In other words, the sensations, characteristics, and quantity of mucus **remain the same each day**. In order to establish if an unchanging pattern of mucus is indeed infertile, you must first observe the same pattern of mucus — same sensation, characteristics, amount — for at least 14 days (two weeks). If *during the postpartum transition* the mucus remains unchanging, the mucus pattern is considered infertile and you are in Phase I. Such a pattern of mucus is called a **Basic Infertile Pattern (BIP)**. It is especially important that you continue to make diligent mucus observations during a BIP. If the mucus changes in quantity, sensations, or characteristics (such as color, quality, spotting or bleeding), then consider the change in the pattern to be Phase II (a fertile time). A return to the BIP signals a return to Phase I. Follow the guideline below to determine when you return to Phase I. **The Couple to Couple League recommends that you discuss this situation with your CCL teacher, who has been specially trained in the BIP, before applying this guideline.**

Basic Infertile Pattern (BIP)

Phase I infertility begins after 14 days (two weeks) of observing and recording mucus and temperature signs AND
- The mucus sensations, characteristics, and quantity remain unchanging AND
- There is no thermal shift

Phase II fertility begins with a change in any of the following: mucus sensations, characteristics, or quantity

Phase I infertility begins again

- On the evening of the fourth day of returning to the BIP AND
- There is no thermal shift

Lochia

There are other vaginal discharges after childbirth that do not indicate fertility, the most obvious of which is lochia. Lochia occurs after childbirth because the uterus is contracting and shrinking back to its pre-pregnancy size and the endometrium is regenerating after the nine months of pregnancy.

For the first few days after childbirth, the lochia is composed mostly of blood, but it may also contain fragments of membranes from the amniotic sac and the coating and fine hair from the baby's skin. The color of this lochia is generally **dark red to brownish** and is called *lochia rubra* (meaning red).

Once blood flow decreases, the discharge becomes **thinner and brownish** in appearance and will contain plasma that oozes from the placental attachment site, white blood cells, and fragments of degenerating endometrium, all of which are part of the normal process of healing and regenerating the uterine lining, so that a future baby could implant on the same site. This lochia is referred to as *lochia serosa*.[1]

At approximately two weeks postpartum, the lochia becomes **thick and white to yellowish** in color and is called *lochia alba* (meaning white). It is composed of mucus (here we are referring to material produced by all epithelial cell layers like the endometrium) and white blood cells. White blood cells color mucus white. Lochia alba continues until three to six weeks postpartum, gradually decreasing in amount.

At this point you may be wondering if you might be confused by the white or yellow discharge (lochia alba), thinking that it might be the start of cervical mucus and the return of fertility. Lochia alba does contain mucus from the endometrium, and so it may have somewhat similar characteristics to cervical mucus, but there are some differences.

First, lochia alba will not produce the type of sensation that cervical mucus produces at the vulva. Second, lochia alba gradually decreases in amount, whereas, cervical mucus that occurs when a woman is ready to ovulate will progressively change, increase in amount, and produce feelings of wetness and slipperiness.

---

[1] Francine Nichols, Ph.D. and Elaine Zwelling, Ph.D., *Maternal-Newborn Nursing — Theory and Practice*, (W.B. Saunders Company, 1997) 980.

Marital intimacy

Marital intimacy takes on a deeper meaning when the newest member of the household is born. Couples learn to re-order their priorities; baby's needs come first as he cannot care for himself. Mom's and Dad's needs come second. A breastfeeding mother must give of herself to provide nourishment; a father must learn to give in other ways like caring for his wife; bathing, rocking, and walking the baby; caring for the other children; and helping around the house. The postpartum household becomes an increasingly self-giving household. Marital intimacy in the presence of abstinence, however, is greatly enhanced when the new mother and father take on these selfless roles. The mature mother knows she is being loved by the selfless acts performed by her husband; the mature father realizes that his wife is caring for their child in the best way possible and that the baby's needs surpass his own for the present.

Postpartum sexual satisfaction

New parents may also need additional insights into achieving satisfaction with their sexual relationships. One problem that can occur during a prolonged phase of infertility, especially with breastfeeding mothers, is an excessively dry vagina because mucus is not being produced. This normally can be overcome in a relaxed, unhurried environment where time is spent lovingly preparing the wife for genital intercourse. With slow and relaxing stimulation, the Bartholin's glands (special glands in the back walls of the vagina), release lubricating fluid to allow for satisfactory intercourse. To be emotionally and physically satisfying, sexual intercourse does not have to be tied to the estrogen production which occurs around ovulation. Rather, it is best tied to the loving touch and consideration between the husband and wife.

Glossary G

Abstinence: The practice of refraining from indulging an appetite or desire, e.g., sexual intercourse.

Amenorrhea: Absence of menstrual periods.

Anovulatory cycle: A menstrual cycle without ovulation.

Antibodies: Proteins that fight infections.

Asthma: A disease of the respiratory system.

Bartholin's glands: Glands in the back walls of the vagina that release lubricating fluid during marital relations.

Basal body temperature: The temperature of the human body at rest or upon awakening, unaffected by food, drink, or activity.

Basic Infertile Pattern (BIP): An unchanging mucus pattern that lasts for at least 14 days in which the sensations, characteristics, and quantity of mucus remain the same each day. This phenomenon sometimes occurs during the postpartum time (or during the premenopausal transition).

Bellagio Consensus Conference on lactational infertility: A conference held in Bellagio, Italy in 1988, in which expert researchers on family planning from around the world tracked the return of fertility in mothers who were not using any method of family planning or fertility awareness while they were exclusively breastfeeding. As a result, they issued a Consensus Statement with regard to exclusive breastfeeding and amenorrhea.

Breakthrough bleeding: A bleeding episode that is not part of menstruation. It can appear as spotting or days of bleeding in the middle of a cycle, and it can also occur as a regular period following an anovulatory cycle. Breakthrough bleeding can mask the presence of mucus, and it can be a potentially fertile time.

Breastfeeding: See continued breastfeeding, exclusive breastfeeding, and mixed breastfeeding.

Cervical mucus: A natural fluid of the body that is necessary for the proper functioning of a woman's reproductive system and is an aid to fertility.

Cervical os: The opening of the cervix.

Cervix: The lower, narrow part of the uterus that extends slightly into the vagina; the opening to the uterus.

Changing mucus pattern: A pattern of mucus in which the mucus sensations and/or characteristics change frequently, but do not disappear.

Colostrum: A yellowish liquid secreted by a mother's breasts for about the first three to five days following childbirth; it is rich in antibodies and contains more protein and minerals, and less sugar and fat, than human breast milk.

Conception: The union of one male sperm and

one female ovum; the beginning of a new human life. Also called fertilization.

Continued breastfeeding: Nursing beyond six months, when the introduction of other foods and liquids are added to complement the breast milk. The baby still nurses and pacifies at the breast on his own schedule.

Continuous mucus: An unusual mucus pattern that is sometimes experienced by breastfeeding mothers; not to be confused with mucus discharge. (See changing mucus pattern, mucus discharge, and unchanging mucus pattern.)

Corpus luteum: A yellow, progesterone-secreting structure that forms from an ovarian follicle after the release of a mature egg. If the egg is not fertilized, the corpus luteum secretes progesterone for approximately 14 days after ovulation.

Diabetes mellitus: A metabolic disorder affecting blood sugar levels; can cause kidney, eye, and nerve damage.

Doering Rule: A formula to determine the infertile time at the beginning of a cycle based on the earliest day of temperature rise in previous cycles. In the absence of mucus, the last day of Phase I infertility is seven days before the earliest first day of temperature rise.

Endometrium: The inner lining of the uterus.

Episiotomy: A surgical incision of the perineum.

Estrogen: A fertility hormone that causes the cervix to undergo physical changes and to secrete mucus, and which causes the development of the endometrium.

Exclusive breastfeeding: Nursing whenever the baby indicates a desire (day or night) during his first six months of life; the baby receives no bottles or early solids, stays near his mother and pacifies at the breast on his own schedule.

Fertile time: The time of a woman's menstrual cycle leading up to and including the time of ovulation, characterized, in part, by the presence of mucus. Sexual intercourse during this time (Phase II) could result in conception.

Fertility: The quality or condition of being able to produce offspring.

Fertilization: The union of one male sperm and one female ovum; the beginning of a new human life. Also called conception.

Follicle: One of thousands of small ovarian sacs

containing an immature ovum; each cycle, one follicle fully matures and is released at ovulation. Upon release of its egg, the follicle becomes a structure called the corpus luteum.

Follicle Stimulating Hormone (FSH): A fertility hormone secreted by the pituitary gland to stimulate the maturation of ovarian follicles.

Formula feeding: A baby is fed with a bottle and receives only milk, ranging from donor milk, to specialty formulas, to cow's milk.

Hemorrhoids: Painful varicose veins in the canal of the anus.

High Temperature Level (HTL): The temperature level that is 0.4° Fahrenheit (0.2° Celsius) above the Low Temperature Level (LTL); used to establish the beginning of Phase III with the Sympto-Thermal Rule.

Hodgkin's disease: A malignant form of lymphoma marked by progressive enlargement of the lymph nodes and spleen and sometimes of the liver.

Hormone: A chemical substance produced by a gland or organ of the body and carried by circulation to other areas where it produces an effect.

Humanae Vitae (On Human Life): Pope Paul VI's 1968 encyclical letter explaining the duty of the transmission of life for married couples.

Hypercholesterolemia: An unusually high level of cholesterol in the blood.

Induced lactation: The process by which a non-pregnant mother is stimulated to lactate.

Infertile time: The time of a woman's menstrual cycle both before the ovulation process begins as well as after ovulation, characterized, in part, by the absence of mucus. Sexual intercourse during these times (Phases I and III) does not result in conception.

Infertility: The quality or condition of being unable to produce offspring.

Lactate: Breastfeed; produce milk.

Lactational amenorrhea: Lack of menstrual periods due to breastfeeding.

Lactational Amenorrhea Method (LAM): A method of family planning based on the high infertility during the first six months postpartum for exclusively breastfeeding mothers in amenorrhea.

Last Dry Day Rule: A formula to determine the

infertile time at the beginning of a cycle based on the appearance of mucus. The end of Phase I is the last day without mucus sensations or characteristics.

Less-fertile mucus: Often described as tacky, sticky, opaque, or thicker than the more-fertile mucus. Less-fertile mucus is usually present both before and after a woman experiences more-fertile mucus leading up to ovulation.

Leukemia: An often fatal cancer in which white blood cells displace normal blood, leading to infection and other disorders.

Lochia: The blood-tinged discharge a woman experiences for about five weeks after childbirth.

Low Temperature Level (LTL): The highest of the normal pre-shift six temperatures. The LTL is the level from which the High Temperature Level (HTL) is determined.

Luteal phase: A stage of the menstrual cycle, lasting about two weeks, from ovulation to the beginning of the next menstrual flow; measured by counting the days from the first day of temperature rise to the last day of the cycle.

Luteinizing Hormone (LH): A fertility hormone produced by the pituitary gland that helps to stimulate ovulation in females.

Lymphoma: A tumor in the lymph node.

Menstruation: The periodic discharge of blood and tissue from the uterus in non-pregnant women from puberty to menopause (following a sustained thermal shift).

Mixed breastfeeding: High mixed: 80% of the feeding comes from the breast; medium mixed: 20–79% of the feeding comes from the breast; low mixed: less than 20% of the feeding comes from the breast.

More-fertile mucus: Mucus that is present during the fertile time prior to ovulation (Phase II) in a woman's menstrual cycle. It is identified by sensations of wetness and/or slipperiness, and/or characteristics that are stretchy, stringy, or resembling raw egg-white.

Mucus characteristics: The qualities of mucus that a woman sees and/or touches when making observations.

Mucus discharge: A discharge that could be the result of an infection; it is generally characterized by an odor and/or unusual type of discharge, which could be irritating or painful.

Mucus patch (patches of mucus): One or more days of mucus sensations/characteristics followed by dry/nothing days without a thermal shift.

Mucus Patch Rule: A rule used to determine the return to Phase I infertility. Phase I infertility returns on the evening of the fourth day of no mucus sensations or characteristics after Peak Day, where Peak Day is the last day of a mucus patch or breakthrough bleeding.

Mucus sensations: The qualities of mucus that a woman feels and senses throughout the day and when wiping at bathroom visits.

Mucus symbols: The graphic symbol used to describe the day's mucus observations: $\bigcirc$ = no mucus, $\ominus$ = less-fertile, $\oplus$ = more-fertile.

Natural Family Planning (NFP): A means of reading a woman's signs of fertility and infertility; also known as fertility awareness.

Non-lactating: Non-breastfeeding; formula feeding.

Ovary: The female reproductive organ containing the ova, or eggs.

Ovulation: The process of an ovarian follicle releasing its ovum, thus making a woman fertile and able to become pregnant.

Ovum: The female reproductive cell, or egg; plural: ova.

Oxytocin: A hormone released from the pituitary gland that stimulates the contraction of the smooth muscles of the uterus during labor, facilitates release of milk during nursing, and assists in postpartum bonding; called the "hormone of love."

Peak Day: The last day of the more-fertile mucus before the drying-up process begins. Peak Day can only be identified in retrospect.

Peak Day in relation to mucus patches and/or breakthrough bleeding: The last day of a mucus patch or breakthrough bleeding.

Perineum: The area between the anus and the front part of the external genitalia in females.

Phase I: A time of infertility, beginning when a woman starts her menstrual bleeding and ending when fertility signs appear.

Phase II: The fertile time of the cycle. It is during this time that the woman ovulates and when conception may occur.

Phase III: The infertile time after ovulation.

Pituitary gland: A gland located at the base of the brain that releases various hormones that control the functions of other organs.

Placenta: The organ inside the uterus that supplies food and oxygen to, and removes waste from, the unborn baby through the umbilical cord.

Postpartum: The term used to explain that a mother has recently given birth and has not yet returned to her pre-pregnancy state.

Postpartum blues: Weepiness or sadness in the early days and weeks after giving birth, resulting from hormonal fluctuations.

Postpartum depression (PPD): Excessive fatigue, insomnia, changes in appetite, difficulty in making decisions, feeling helpless, negative attitudes, and thoughts of death or suicide; usually highly treatable.

Postpartum urinary incontinence: Temporary incontinence (inability to control bladder) during the early weeks after childbirth.

Pre-shift six: Six lower temperatures immediately preceding at least three temperatures that rise above them in a sustained pattern; used to set the Low Temperature Level (LTL).

Progesterone: A fertility hormone secreted by the corpus luteum that prepares the uterus for the fertilized ovum and helps sustain a pregnancy.

Prolactin: Called "the mothering hormone," it aids in the accelerated growth of breast tissue during pregnancy. With suckling, prolactin levels increase and the hormone stimulates and maintains the secretion of milk, and enables natural bonding between mother and baby.

Responsible parenthood: The virtuous decisions by a married couple to plan or to postpone conception through the knowledge and practice of fertility awareness.

Seminal residue: Seminal fluid that sometimes remains in a woman's vaginal area after she has sexual intercourse.

Shortest-Cycle Rule: A formula to determine the infertile time at the beginning of a woman's menstrual cycle based on previous cycle history lengths. In the last 12 cycles: if the shortest cycle is 26 days or more, she assumes infertility on Cycle Days 1 through 6; if the shortest cycle is less than 26 days, she assumes infertility on the cycle days preceding her previous shortest cycle minus 20. (For application when cycle history is lacking or when coming off birth control hormones, see page 4.)

Suckle: To feed from the breast.

Sympto-Thermal Method (STM): A method of fertility awareness that utilizes the observation of changes in the cervical mucus, basal body temperature, and cervix to determine the fertile and infertile times of a woman's menstrual cycle.

Sympto-Thermal Rule: A formula to determine the infertile time of a woman's menstrual cycle following ovulation. Phase III begins on the evening of the third day of drying-up after Peak Day combined with three normal post-peak temperatures in a rising pattern above the LTL, AND the third temperature at or above the HTL, OR the cervix closed and hard for three days. If the previous conditions are not met, then Phase III begins after waiting an additional post-peak day for another temperature above the LTL.

Temperatures in a rising pattern: Three consecutive temperature readings that are higher than the six preceding readings. These do not have to be successively higher, but it is essential that each reading — considered individually — is higher than each one of the six lower readings; used to interpret the temperature sign.

Thermal shift: At least three temperatures that are higher than the six preceding temperatures; used to calculate the Sympto-Thermal Rule and Temperature-Only Rule.

Unchanging mucus pattern: A mucus pattern experienced by some breastfeeding mothers in which the mucus sensations, characteristics and quantity remain the same each day; could appear right after the lochia ends or later, sometimes for a period of time.

Urinary incontinence: The inability to keep urine in the bladder.

Uterus: A hollow, pear-shaped organ in which a baby grows during the nine months of pregnancy; frequently called the womb.

Vagina: The female genital canal extending from the uterus to the vulva.

Index

Induced lactation, 13, 68

Infant mortality rate, 14

Infection, 38

Infertile time, 68

Infertility, 68; natural, 9, 15

Insomnia, 12

International & American Associations of Clinical Nutritionists, 63

International Journal of Obstetrics and Gynecology, 20

K

Kennedy, K., 19–20

Key measurable signs, 21–23, 29, 38–39

Kracht, Linda, 13, 62

L

Labbok, M., 19–20

Lactate, 13, 68

Lactating, 17

Lactational amenorrhea, 9, 68; length of, 17; while exclusively breastfeeding, 16

Lactational Amenorrhea Method (LAM), 20, 68

Lancet, 19

Last Dry Day Rule, 4, 68

Lauwers, J., 14, 16

Lawrence, Robert, 22

Lawrence, Ruth, 22

Less-fertile mucus, 69

Let-down reflex, 10, 15

Letters of C. S. Lewis, 49

Leukemia, 15, 69

Lewis, C.S., 49

Lochia, 9, 23–24, 36, 41, 65, 69; alba, 65; rubra, 65; serosa, 65

Low mixed breastfeeding, 18

Low Temperature Level (LTL), 69

Luteal phase, 38, 69

Luteinizing Hormone (LH), 8–9, 27, 69

Lymphoma, 15, 69

M

Main NFP course, 7

Marital intimacy, 49, 66

Marital relations, 4, 28, 39

Maternal-Newborn Nursing — Theory and Practice,
65

McNeilly, A., 19

Medium mixed breastfeeding, 18

Menstruation, 3, 69

Mixed breastfeeding, 17–18, 69; and return of fertility, 18; high, 18; low, 18; medium, 18

Mood swings, 11

More-fertile mucus, 69

Mucus, 23; absent, 29; changing pattern, 37–38; continuous, 29, 36–37, 64, 68; following breakthrough bleeding, 34; patches, 29–30, 69; Patches of Mucus Practice Chart, 31, 58; same as during pre-pregnancy cycles, 29; unchanging pattern, 36; when breastfeeding, 29; when formula feeding, 23; with bleeding, 29; with spotting, 29

Mucus characteristics, 69

Mucus discharge, 69

Mucus observations, when breastfeeding, 28; when first learning, 23, 28

Mucus patch, 29–30, 69; Practice Chart, 31, 58

Mucus Patch Rule, 30, 34, 41, 69; and temperature rise, 30

Mucus sensations, 69

Mucus symbols, 69

N

National Resource Defense Council, 12

Natural Conception Regulation, 23

Natural Family Planning (NFP), vii, 47, 69; in the postpartum time, 49

Natural spacing, 48

NFP-supportive physicians, 62

Nichols, Ph.D., Francine, 65

Non-injectable hormonal birth control, 4

Non-lactating, 69

Non-lactating mother, and return of fertility, 22

Not on consecutive days, 28

Nutrition, 11–12, 63

Nutritional response testing, 63

O

Obesity, 15

One More Soul, 62

On Human Life, 48

Osteoporosis, 15

Ovarian cancer, 15

Ovary, 37, 69

Overweight, 15